Save Your Life

With the Phenomenal Lemon (& Lime!)

Becoming pH Balanced in an Unbalanced World

by

Blythe Ayne, Ph.D.

Save Your Life

With the Phenomenal Lemon (& Lime!)

Becoming pH Balanced in an Unbalanced World

by

Blythe Ayne, Ph.D.

Save Your Life
With the Phenomenal Lemon (& Lime!)
Becoming Balanced in an Unbalanced World
Blythe Ayne, Ph.D.

Emerson & Tilman, Publishers
129 Pendleton Way #55
Washougal, WA 98671

Book & cover design by Blythe Ayne
All Text & Graphics
© Blythe Ayne

Other books in the *How to Save Your Life* series:
Save Your Life with the Power of pH Balance
Save Your Life with the Elixir of Water
Save Your Life with Stupendous Spices

www.BlytheAyne.com

Save Your Life with with the Phenomenal Lemon (& Lime)!
Becoming Balanced in an Unbalanced World

ebook ISBN: 978-1-947151-06-2
Paperback ISBN: 978-1-947151-07-9
Large Print ISBN: 978-1-947151-67-3
Hardback ISBN: 978-1-947151-05-5

[1. HEALTH & FITNESS/Diet & Nutrition/Nutrition
2. HEALTH & FITNESS/Healing
3. HEALTH & FITNESS/Diseases/General]
BIC: FM
Second Edition

Table of Contents:

With gratitude to T. Traviskas & C. Greear for their editorial assistance.

Save Your Life
With the Phenomenal Lemon & Lime
Becoming pH Balanced in an Unbalanced World

> *"(You) do not live off the food you eat*
> *but off of the energy that is produced*
> *from the food you eat."*
> A.F. Beddoe,
> ***Biological Ionization in Human Nutrition***

Introduction:

If you've never particularly thought about lemons and limes, you may be astounded by some of what you're about to read. What's more important, when you put the following easy-to-accomplish, easy-to-understand suggestions and information into practice, you and your loved ones will experience improved health, heightened emotional well-being, and increased longevity.

A Brief Overview

Let's take a quick look at the benefits that are possible from fresh lemons and limes:

Freshly squeezed lemon and lime juice has antibacterial, antiseptic, anti-inflammatory, antiviral, anti-fungal, and antihistamine properties. It has also shown antibiotic effects. It fights infections and helps in the production of white blood cells and antibodies in the blood, which attack invading microorganisms. Their antioxidant property destroys roving free radicals, preventing cardiovascular disease, stroke, cancers, and a myriad other health issues.

By supporting the proper metabolism of cells, they are prevented from becoming carcinogenic. One of the positive processes of the components of lemons and limes is to interfere with the formation of the carcinogenic chemical compounds known as nitro-samines in the gut. The digestive system is where eighty percent of your immune system resides, so having the health-sustaining components found in lemons and limes hard at work in the gut is a signifi-cant contributor to great health.

Lemon and lime juice can reduce the symptoms of colds, flu, fever, throat infections, indigestion, con-stipation, diarrhea, colic pain, gastric problems, rickets, internal bleeding, burns, scurvy, peptic ulcer, fatigue, weak eyes, and tooth and gum prob-lems. Lemon and lime juice lowers cholesterol, reduces phlegm in the body, purifies the blood, controls bleeding, helps dissolve pancreatic stones, gallstones and kidney stones.

Lemons and limes reduce the symptoms of arthritis, inflammatory polyarthritis, osteoarthritis, and all the other "itises" as well as sciatica. The healthful components of lemons and limes clear out calcium deposits, the painful factor in gout, by neutralizing the high uric acid levels in the blood.

Lemons and limes are effectively used in the treatment of cholera, tuberculosis, malaria, diphtheria, diabetes, cancers, heart disease, arteriosclerosis, high blood pressure, allergies, asthma, and other respiratory problems.

The high level of potassium in lemons and limes nourishes nerve and brain cells, thereby improving nerve and brain function.

In utero, lemons and limes contribute to the making of strong bones in the developing baby.

Lemons and limes are used for general eye care, dental care, skincare, and hair care. These brightly-colored fruit can improve appetite and, last but certainly not least in this impressive—and still not exhaustive!—list of benefits is that lemons and limes can significantly contribute to weight loss.

In addition, adding lemon or lime juice or slices to your glass of water increases the effect of water's hydration of your body.

Before delving into yet more amazing details of these far-reaching benefits, let's take a brief historical look at lemons and limes to see, among other interesting facts, how they came to be readily accessible to those of us who live in northern climes, which are inhospitable to the growth of citrus.

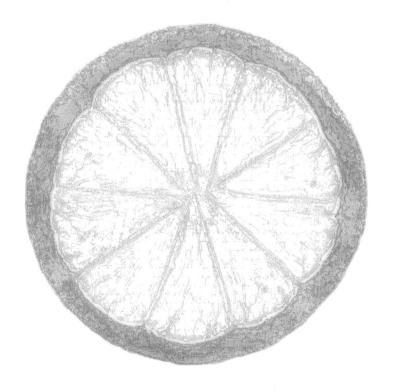

Chapter 1:
Ancient History to Modern Times

*"Your health is what you make of it.
Everything you do and think either adds to
the vitality, energy and spirit you possess
or takes away from it."*

Ann Wigmore,

The Hippocrates Diet and Health Program

Question: Which came first, the lemon or the lime?
No fair peeking ....
Answer: The citron

First Came the Citron

The scientific name of the citron, Citrus *medica*, is derived from its ancient name, *Median apple*. This is not a reference to medical usage, although historically it had—and still has—several medical applications.

Media was the ancient name for Persia, and the citron has also been called the Persian Apple.

Citron is the fruit of a small, thorny evergreen tree that grows 8 to 15 feet tall, native to India and Southeast Asia. The fruit of the citron looks lemon-like, but is larger, has a thick, fragrant rind and not much pulp.

Although the fruit straight off the tree is not edible, as mentioned, it was discovered in ancient times to have important medical applications. The citron was used to cure or improve intestinal problems, seasickness, and added to wine as an antidote to poison. The outer rind was used as an antibiotic.

The evergreen citron bears fruit year-round. At any given time it will have flowers, ripening fruit, and fully ripe fruit on its branches all at once, and in this manner it continually produces fruit.

The citron is identified as a very old and "original species." Its molecular structure provides evidence that all our other cultivated citrus came from developing hybrids of the citron, along with the mandarin, pomelo, and papeda. The citron is regarded as the purest fruit, as it is fertilized by self-pollination.

Lemons

Lemons (*Citrus limon*), which grow on a small ever-green tree, are believed to have been first developed in Southern India, Burma or China thousands of years ago, although its origins are lost in the mystery of time. Lemons are variously reported as a hybrid between the lime and the citron, or the sour orange and citron.

The first appearance of lemons in written history (discovered to date) was in a 10th-century Arabic volume on farming. The lovely lemon tree was also used as an ornamental plant in Islamic gardens. Arabs then brought lemons to North Africa and Spain in the 11th century.

The origin of the word *"lemon"* is probably Middle Eastern, from Arabic and Persian *limun*. In a 1420 Middle English customs document the word "lemon" occurs, and may well be the first English recording of the word.

The Crusaders discovered lemons in Palestine. They brought them back to Europe, and subsequently, in 1493, Christopher Columbus brought them to the New World, where they've grown in Florida ever since.

In the mid-1700s, seamen had profoundly vitamin C deficient diets and were dying at sea from scurvy. Sometimes the majority of the crew would die, with ships returning to home ports virtual ghost ships.

At the time, Dr. James Lind experimented with putting lemon juice in some of the sailors' diets, even though there was no concept of vitamin C—nor a concept of *any* vitamin, for that matter. Although he wasn't the first to believe that citrus was somehow a cure for scurvy, he was the first doctor to run a clinical experiment to investigate his theory. This experiment is one of the first recorded formal experiments in the history of medicine.

Jump ahead another one-hundred years, and we see lemons playing a role in the California Gold Rush in the mid-1800s. The scurvy-preventing, vitamin C-loaded fruit was so needed by sun-deprived miners that they would pay as much as one dollar for one lemon, the equivalent of $29.50 in current prices.

Limes

The two species of limes that are most common are the Persian lime (*Citrus latifolia*) and the Key lime (*Citrus aurantiifolia*).

The Persian lime, first grown commercially in Iraq (historically, Persia), is wonderfully fragrant, seedless and larger than the Key lime. Because hurricane Andrew nearly wiped out the Florida Persian lime orchards in 1992, Persian limes are now primarily imported from Mexico. Persian limes are hardier than Key limes, with a longer shelf life.

We are familiar with the lime's bright green color, but they will turn yellow if allowed to fully ripen.

The Key lime derives its name from growing in the Florida Keys. It's a beautiful tree with leaves that resemble orange tree leaves. In fact, its scientific name, *aurantiifolia*, relates to its resemblance to the leaves of the orange tree (*Citrus aurantium*).

The word "lime" derives from both French and Arabic, "*lim*." Limes grow in tropical and subtropical climate. They bear fruit all year long and thus provide a nearly continual harvest. Their "migration" is similar to lemons, having been brought by Arab traders from Asia to Northern Africa and Egypt in the 10th century.

Subsequently, the Moors took limes to Spain during the 13th century. From there the Crusaders carried the lime throughout southern Europe, where they grew in the southernmost regions.

Christopher Columbus brought limes, along with lemons, to the New World, where they were planted in the favorable hot, humid environment of the Caribbean countries. When, several hundred years later, the British traders and explorers took advantage of the limes that grew in the West Indies British colonies to prevent scurvy, they acquired the still occasionally used nickname "Limey."

Limes finally came to the United States in the 1500s, when the Spanish explorers brought the lime that was successfully growing in the West Indies to the Florida Keys. During the 1600s, Spanish missionaries tried to plant lime trees in California, but their efforts were not successful, as the California climate couldn't support the Key lime.

Then, during the California Gold Rush, the lime was also, just like the lemon, in great demand by miners. Because of this demand, limes were imported from Mexico and Tahiti.

The nutritional benefits of limes are not significantly different from lemons. They are both excellent sources of vitamin C, B vitamins, potassium, folic acid, enzymes, biophotons, the phytochemical flavonoids, and other components. (Please check out the glossary in the back of the book if any of the multi-syllabic tongue twisters you encounter in the book are unfamiliar to you.)

For an in-depth look at lemon and lime nutrition and their chemical components, see Chapter 7: *What's in These Lovely Fruits to make them so Potent?*

CHAPTER HIGH POINTS:

1. Lemons were first developed as a hybrid between the citron and other citrus fruits, thousands of years ago in the Far East.

2. Important medical applications of the citron have been employed since before the dawn of history.

3. The Crusaders and Arabs brought the fruit to Africa and Europe from the 10th to the 13th centuries, and Christopher Columbus brought them to the New World in 1493.

4. Lemons and limes were believed to prevent scurvy in the 1700s by Dr. James Lind, even though the concept of vitamins had not yet been imagined.

5. Miners in the mid-1800s Gold Rush paid as much as $1 for a lemon, equivalent to $29.50 in today's dollars, in order to prevent scurvy.

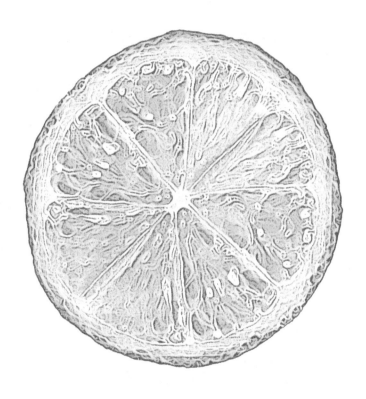

Chapter 2:
The Many Wonderful Health Benefits of Lemons & Limes

"Raw food brings longevity and life force into your body. Hormones, oxygen, phytochemicals and enzymes are kaput (after cutting a fruit or vegetable) in 15 minutes."

Dr. Brian Clement

Let's jump right into the numerous and remarkable health benefits of lemons and limes, and their various applications. This includes everything from aromatherapy to their being used as an effective complementary treatment for serious disease.

The three components of lemon—1. the peel or rind, 2. the pith or albedo, and 3. the segmented flesh—have been used for thousands of years in the oldest medical traditions, namely, East Indian Ayurvedic, East Indian Siddha, and traditional Chinese medicines.

These ancient traditions, from the past and into the present, have a frontline commitment to prevention first, as well as fully-developed treatments for active illnesses, diseases and disorders.

One of the most important facts regarding lemons and ~ limes is that, although they are acidic in their base form, *they are alkaline-forming in the human body.* Water with fresh squeezed lemon or lime in it increases the body's alkalinity.

In the 1. contaminated environment, 2. emotionally stressful, 3. poor diet world we live in—three factors that contribute to your body becoming more acidic— we need all the alkalizing help we can get. Drinking a glass of lemon or lime water before a meal will help your body alkalize to attain a balanced pH.

However, it is better to drink your lemon or lime water half-an-hour to an hour before a meal, as it can more fully do its work. A slightly alkaline body keeps you healthy and able to ward off illness and disease.

The significant amount of Vitamin C in lemons and limes strengthens the immune system. Their antibacterial properties contribute to controlling the decomposition of tissue and the growth of pathogenic bacteria.

Some of the most beneficial components of lemons and limes are their biophotons (measurable sunlight energy) and their live enzymes. The antioxidant properties of lemons and limes come from their amazing phytochemicals. These are potent detoxifiers that protect you against bacteria with their anti-biotic effect. The phytochemicals maximize enzyme functioning and they oxygenate the body.

Lemons and limes are an excellent, natural and healthy means to boost your immune system, and a strong defense in staving off infections. Their antibacterial attribute destroys bacteria in the mouth and in the gut, even as they alkalize your system.

Calcium deposits are one of the body's major culprits, hardening arteries, developing gout and all the other types of arthritis, and forming kidney stones, pancreatic stones and gallstones. Lemon and lime juice contributes to the presence of urinary citrate, which can reverse *and even prevent* the mineral crystallization buildup of calcium deposits.

A body becomes overly acidic from one or more of the following:

- free radical damage
- emotional stress
- physical stress
- accumulation of toxins
- legal and street drugs
- alcohol
- tobacco
- junk food

The body's defense system will then pull the alkaline minerals—calcium, magnesium, and phosphorus—

from teeth and bones to buffer the acids in order to keep the blood alkaline.

Here's a boggling fact. The Centers of Disease Control and Prevention have reported that Americans have 116 synthetic compounds in their bodies! Your body will use fresh lemon and lime juice to cleanse your entire system of these myriad impurities.

Search & Destroy Mission

Lemon and lime juice have the seemingly miraculous ability to search and destroy those harmful components that hide out in joints, organs and tissues, piling up—unbeknownst to us—until one day they reach a critical mass and create pain and disease.

As mentioned above, lemons and limes are acidic in their base form. Disease process is acidic. How can something that is acidic battle something that is acidic? This is the part that is mysterious and fascinating: although a lemon or a lime is *acidic*, it has the interesting property of burning as *alkaline* ash in the human body, thereby getting to places where the destructive acidic components are, and then destroying them by burning off as alkaline. It neutralizes the area.

Think of fresh lemon or lime juice as on a covert mission—it invades the enemy camp (overly acidic site) dressed as the enemy (acidic), and then whips off the enemy uniform (burns as alkaline ash) and saves the homeland—namely you! Or your child, or your parent, or another loved one.

Our bodies and our earth must be in pH balance to be healthy. Disease process is a process of being excessively acidic. A slightly alkaline state is an inhospitable environment for disease, and the disease will "die." The juice from a fresh lemon or lime—or even half a lemon or lime—every day contributes significantly to alkalizing your body.

What's particularly fantastic about all the wonders of drinking a cup of room temperature water with fresh lemon or lime juice squeezed into it is that it's not contraindicated by other treatments or medications. Lemons and limes are fruit. You can be on your medications, on your health program, under a doctor's care, and drink lemon or lime juice. You have nothing to lose, and perhaps much to gain by simply including this daily habit. Why not start now?

Caution: People on blood thinners, please discuss your daily consumption of lemon and/or lime juice with your health care professional. Also, lemon/lime consumption is contraindicated, of course, for the few rare individuals who are allergic to citrus.

NOTE: There are a few cautions throughout the book. These can also be found together in the back of the book under Chapter 8 entitled *Concerns & Cautions*. There are only a few, and they are minimal in scope.

Simple Experiment

If you're still saying, "I don't believe it," try this simple experiment sometime if you have heartburn (many people do because many people are acidic). Rather than reach for the antacid, squeeze a couple of tablespoons of fresh lemon juice into a glass of room temperature water and drink it. You'll be surprised to discover your heartburn abates in a few minutes, and may completely disappear.

Do you ever wake up in the middle of the night with that alcohol or sugar or salty (or all three) late-in-the-evening indulgence clawing its way back up your throat? Drink a mug of slightly warm water with fresh lemon juice squeezed into it, then lie partially elevated, and you'll soon be back in the land of nod.

However, to avoid the interruption of your sleep because of indigestion, be attentive to what you consume in the late evening. Your body does not appreciate having to process highly acidic materials when it's busy working to rejuvenate you during sleep. Alcohol, sugar and excessive salt (potato chips, etc.) are extremely acidic.

A bit of fresh lemon or lime juice in warm water in the evening is a good tonic. But keep in mind that straight lemon or lime juice can be harmful to tooth enamel, so be sure to follow it with a glass of room temperature water.

Caution: Straight lemon or lime juice can be harmful to tooth enamel. Always mix the juice with water.

CHAPTER HIGH POINTS:

1. The components of lemon—the peel or rind, pith or albedo, and segmented flesh—have been used for thousands of years in the oldest medical traditions to make people well.

2. One of the most important facts regarding lemons and limes is that, although they are acidic in their base form, they are alkaline-forming in the human body. Water with fresh squeezed lemon or lime in it increases the body's alkalinity.

3.　1. Contaminated environment

　　2. Emotional stress

　　3. Poor diet

contribute to a person becoming more acidic.

4. Phytochemicals are antioxidant detoxifiers that protect against bacteria.

5. Calcium deposits are one of the body's major culprits.

6. An acidic body pulls the alkaline minerals—calcium, magnesium, phosphorus—from teeth and bones to keep the blood alkaline.

7. Americans have 116 synthetic compounds in their bodies.

8. Our bodies and the earth must be in pH balance to be alive.

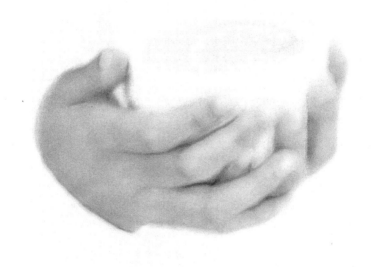

Chapter 3:
Specific Health Effects

"You have a choice. You can continue eating foods manufacturers want you to buy that are making you unhealthy. Or you can return to eating the foods God provided for you, already magnificently packaged in their own skins, rinds, pods, and shells, foods that contain all the human-appropriate vitamins and minerals you need, and the right proportion of sugar, fat, salt and calories."

Rabbi Celso Cukierkorn
The Miracle Diet: Lose Weight, Gain Health

Let's investigate in more detail how lemons and limes affect particular bodily systems, diseases, and disorders to improve your health.

Lemons & Limes & Gastrointestinal Tract—Digestion

Lemons and limes have an amazing ability to assist your body in its digestive and elimination processes, supporting digestion and preventing various digestive problems such as heartburn, constipation, nausea, and parasites, while relieving the unpleasant side effects of bloating and eructations. Why is this? Because, interestingly, both lemons and limes have an atomic structure similar to the human body's own components of hydrochloric acid, bile, and saliva.

This means that lemon and lime juice can, *and does—* at a level of effectiveness that is virtually unique among everything that is edible!—break down and eliminate all the body does not need and that compromises your health.

A glass of room-temperature lemon or lime water first thing in the morning has been an East Indian Yogic, Ayurvedic (East Indian medicine) ritual for hundreds, if not thousands, of years. It was and is used for stimulating digestion and eliminating what Ayurveda refers to as *ama*, the toxic slime that builds up in the GI (gastrointestinal) tract.

Drinking a glass of fresh-squeezed lemon or lime juice in room temperature (not hot, not cold) water liquefies bile, while, at the same time, aids in the control of excess bile. Lemon or lime juice alleviates, and in many cases eliminates, diarrhea and constipation, and lime reduces nausea when a piece of it, including the rind, is chewed and swallowed.

The aroma of lemons and limes makes the mouth water. In fact, even the *thought* of biting a lemon or lime makes the mouth water, as yours may be doing right now, reading this. This mouth-watering is an essential process in digestion. This starts the enzymes to break down the food into usable components and is the first line of defense to assure your excellent health, your perfect weight, and your emotional well-being.

Saliva begins to digest your food so that your whole body can put it to its best use. When the attending acids break down the food into usable components of macromolecules, the flavonoids (you will find more about flavonoids under **Lemons & Limes & Anticancer Properties**) stimulate the digestive system, triggering increased secretion of bile, acids, and digestive juices to extract the optimum absorption of nutrients, and to stimulate peristaltic motion. Peristaltic motion is the involuntary constriction and relaxation of the muscles of the intestine, moving the food contents forward on the body's conveyor belt.

When you picture this, doesn't it make you want to assure that every single component that's on the conveyor belt in your digestive system is the absolute best component it can possibly be? No faulty factory returns here—you produce only the best!

Because East Indians and neighboring countries, in their inimitable and ancient wisdom, know the value of lemons and limes to essential health, they also usually have lemon pickle with lunch and dinner.

Enzymes for a Healthy Liver

Every single toxin that comes into your body must ultimately be processed by the liver before it can be removed. Until the liver can get to toxins to do its job, the toxins are stored in fat cells. Ultimately, the liver converts all toxins, these harmful chemicals, into water-soluble molecules that the body then eliminates. If the liver becomes congested with toxic overload, the toxins remain in fat cells, making it virtually impossible to lose body fat. It also increases the risk for disease processes to get a foothold.

If you drink a glass of room temperature fresh-squeezed lemon or lime water first thing in the morning, it stimulates the liver to produce bile, which breaks down lipids—that is to say, fats. This, in turn, contributes to the thorough digestion of foods. The components of lemon or lime juice clear the liver of toxins.

How this works is that the liver uses fresh lemon or lime juice to make enzymes. It then uses these enzymes to perform its filtering functions. Interestingly, it has been shown that fresh lemon or lime juice can be used by the liver for enzyme production *more effectively than any other food.*[1]

The enzymes assist in the digestion of unhealthy amounts of fat, salt, sugar, and food additives—all of which compromise the overall health of the body. Enzymes also assist in eliminating these unhealthy components from your system, as well as assisting in their absorption, to assure that the nutritional value gets to where it's needed.

Lemon and lime juice also helps the blood oxygen levels by adjusting the calcium and oxygen levels of the liver when regulating the blood carbohydrates.

Citric acid, which is the number one carrier of bio-chemicals in the body, is an outstanding chelator (a molecule that binds to another, usually larger, molecule), and can form soluble complexes with calcium. This process is significant, for example, in dissolving pancreatic stones and kidney stones.

Lemons & Limes for Maximum Kidney & Urinary System Function

Lemon and lime juice stimulates and cleanses the kidneys, and their juice contributes to forming urinary citrate. Urinary citrate has the ability to prevent or reverse dietary mineral crystallization— that is to say, prevent and even cure kidney stones, according to the American Urological Association.[2]

Lemons and limes have a particularly high potassium content, this potassium removes the precipitates and toxic substances that have been deposited in the kidneys and the bladder.

The juice of lemons and limes also acts as a disinfectant and, as such, helps the body cure infections in the urinary system. This process removes the calcium deposits in the urinary tract, clearing the blockage of urine, and even contributes to stopping prostate growth.

Lemons & Limes—Keep Your Gallbladder!

Lemon liquefies bile. This interferes with the ability of gallstones to form. Furthermore, drinking lemon juice with olive oil breaks up gallstones that already exist.

Don't wait until you have a full-on gallbladder attack. A habit of daily lemon juice is a great preventative.

If you're having occasional discomfort with your gallbladder, you have a "stiff," uncomfortable sensation generally on your right side, but sometimes radiating to the left along the bra line, begin a regimen of a couple of tablespoons of fresh-squeezed lemon juice with a tablespoon of extra virgin olive oil in the morning, every morning.

My mother's doctor told her seven years ago that she ought to have her gallbladder removed. My mother began the above practice, lemon juice and extra virgin olive oil every day, and still has her gallbladder—no pain or discomfort and symptom-free.

Ask people who have had their gallbladder removed what that's like. They will give you a list of discomforts that, had they had their lemon juice and olive oil, they may not have had to suffer.

The gallbladder *is the only organ in the body that stores fluid to aid with digestion.* It stores the bile made by the liver. The gallbladder also helps digest nutrients and assists in removing cholesterol and toxins. It emulsifies and breaks down fats so they're more easily digested. All the other organs, and in particular the liver, must take up the slack if the gallbladder has been removed.

Caution: DO NOT IGNORE gallbladder discomfort. You MUST get medical attention for your gallbladder issues. A ruptured gallbladder is life-threatening, and if a gallbladder ruptures, it must be removed. The above remedy is for prevention—continue to work in concert with your medical professional to keep your gallbladder in tip-top shape.

Lesser Caution: Although there are many benefits to eating the peel of lemons and limes, they do contain oxalates, and oxalates can crystallize. People who tend to have kidney stones, pancreatic stones or gallstones should probably avoid eating lemon or lime peels, or foods made with lemon or lime zest from the rinds.

Lemons & Limes Positively Affect Hypertension & Heart Health

Lemon and lime water normalizes blood. If blood is too thin, the juice will help it improve its coagulation to a normal range. If it is too thick and/or sticky, the lemon/lime water will help it become more free-flowing.

Lemon and lime water assists the body in being appropriately alkaline. The blood is waging a battle against acidity when it is too thick or too thin. However, if you are on warfarin, work closely with your health care professional regarding drinking lemon or lime juice.

Blood pressure is the amount of force against the walls of arteries as the heart pumps the blood through the body. If your blood vessels are constricted because they are not healthy, this drives blood pressure up.

High blood pressure takes a toll on fragile blood vessels, is taxing on the heart, hard on the entire system, and can cause heart attacks and strokes. The high potassium content in lemons and limes has been scientifically linked to stabilizing blood pressure. It provides the nervous system with clear pathways to assure that it sends steady signals to the heart, and thus your heart health is improved.

One major factor driving high blood pressure is not drinking enough water. The lack of adequate water, that is to say, forcing your body to endure the experience of long term, chronic dehydration, contributes to high blood pressure because inadequate watering of the human body causes blood vessels to constrict. Every cell in your body is composed largely of water, and if there's not enough of it, the vessels essentially shrivel up. They constrict.

When you drank enough water when you were healthy, your blood flowed happily along its many wide, clean, open river banks. Then, with the habit of inadequate water, these river banks closed in, and now your poor blood is trying to make its way along shriveled, muddy little stream beds.

And people wonder why they have high blood pressure!

If you have high blood pressure, you *MUST* drink adequate water *every single day*. It is a necessity for good health and longevity.

The minimum amount of water to drink daily is one-half your body weight in ounces (for example, if you weigh 150 pounds, then daily drink 75 ounces of water, but, even if you weigh less, do not drink less than eight 8-ounce glasses). Lemons or limes in the water add potassium and help the body absorb the water. Plus the water tastes more inviting!

You'll discover that once you establish this habit you'll crave your lemon or lime water every day. Potassium regulates blood pressure, which prevents nausea and dizziness, and this, in turn, contributes to feeling relaxed in mind and body, reducing depression and emotional stress.

Lemons & Limes Impressive Anticancer Properties

Lemons and limes contain plant pigments known as flavonoid compounds. These compounds are called limonoids and limonene. Limonoids, found in the segments and albedo of lemons and limes, and limonene, found in the rind, are phytochemical (*phyto* is Greek for "plant") compounds.

These are disease-fighting compounds so potent that they've been shown to modify viruses and carcinogens and can even induce cancer cell death. The flavonoids have antioxidant, anticancer, antiallergic, anti-inflammatory, anti-microbial and anti-diarrheal properties.

So far, they appear to be particularly beneficial for protecting against skin, breast, stomach, mouth, lung, and colon cancers.[3] (Nutrition and Cancer, 2001).

Limonene has anti-cancer properties that help to increase the level of specific enzymes that detoxify carcinogens.

Naringenin is also found in the skins of lemons and limes. It is a rich antioxidant, free radical scavenger, and anti-inflammatory flavanone that minimizes cancer development, promotes carbohydrate metabolism, and modulates the immune system. It not only helps prevent damage to DNA but, stunningly, even *repairs* DNA.

Limonins are extremely bioavailable, which is why citrus limonoids are particularly potent anti-carcinogens, preventing cancerous cells from proliferating.

The US Agricultural Research Service (ARS) ran an experiment that demonstrated how the human body readily absorbs and utilizes long-acting limonin. Limonin is attached to a glucose (sugar) molecule, the body easily digests the compound, cleaving off the sugar molecule and releasing the limonin.

There were sixteen volunteers in the ARS experiment. Each was given limonin glucoside in varying amounts. What they discovered was that limonin was still in the plasma of all subjects, except the one who received the least amount, after six hours, and traces remained present in five of the volunteers 24 hours later.

Other natural anti-carcinogens, such as the phenols in green tea and chocolate, are also very bioavailable but are only present for four to six hours.

Several other fascinating research studies have shown that cell cycles—including whether a cell will divide, called mitosis, or die, called apoptosis—are favorably altered by lime juice. Also, the activities of the immune system white blood cells called monocytes have been shown to be positively affected by lime juice.

Monocytes, half of which are stored in the spleen, are the largest corpuscles in the blood. They can move quickly to infections where they divide and differentiate into dendritic cells and macrophages to bring about an immune response.

Lemons & Limes Get the Gout Out!

Gout, a type of arthritis, is caused by an accumulation of free radicals and uric acid. When uric acid builds up in blood, tissues, and urine, then crystallizes in the joints, it causes inflammation and pain. Most commonly in toes and feet, gout may also appear in small hand joints, the heel of the hand, ankles, knees, elbows, wrists, or an ear. It is accompanied by swelling, inflammation and intense pain.

This is caused by the chemicals known as purines as they metabolize. When they metabolize, they become uric acid. It's the job of the digestive enzyme uricase to break down the purines, but people with gout are overly acidic and have inadequate uricase, which is alkaline, to break down the purines.

The problem can become considerably more severe than a painful toe, however, as continued excess uric acid can cause kidney stones, kidney disease, and, worst scenario, kidney failure.

Lemons and limes, with their plenteous detoxifiers and antioxidants in flavonoids and vitamin C, detoxify the body, blocking and destroying free radicals. Lemon and lime juice dissolves uric acid (as well as other acidic impurities), resulting in abatement of joint pain. It gets the gout out! It also takes the sting out of other inflammatory disorders and is effective in abating (or eliminating) arthritis, rheumatism, and sciatica.

Lemons & Limes Abate Arthritis, Rheumatoid Arthritis, Polyarthritis, Osteoarthritis & All the Other Itises

Scientific studies have shown that vitamin C-rich lemons and limes, with their anti-inflammatory, detoxifying and alkalizing processes, provide us with powerful protection against painful, inflammatory rheumatoid arthritis, including polyarthritis, osteoarthritis, and rheumatism.

Free radicals that interact with healthy cells, damaging them and their membranes and causing inflammation and painful swelling, are stopped in their tracks by the powerhouse of vitamin C. Lemons and limes are also diuretic and further help to treat rheumatism and arthritis by expediting the flushing of toxins and bacteria out of the body.

The *Annals of the Rheumatic Diseases*[4] conducted a study of more than 20,000 subjects. All the participants were initially arthritis-free at the beginning of the study. They all kept diet diaries. The study compared the participants who developed inflammatory polyarthritis with those who did not.

The results were unambiguous. The subjects who consumed the least amount of vitamin C-rich foods were *more than three times more likely to develop arthritis* than the subjects who consumed the highest amounts of vitamin C!

It's recommended for anyone who suffers from any of the nearly one-hundred forms of arthritis, to drink one or two ounces of fresh-squeezed lemon or lime juice (at least ½ of a lemon or a whole lime), diluted in a cup (more or less, suited to preference) of room temperature water, half-an-hour to an hour before every meal and at bedtime.

The Positive Effect of Lemons & Limes on Diabetes

The high vitamin content of lemons and limes helps to stabilize blood sugar levels. Blood sugars have been shown to lower when drinking lemon or lime juice shortly before or with meals.

Since free radicals can damage blood vessels and can change cholesterol to make it more likely to build up in artery walls, vitamin C is helpful in preventing the development of diabetic heart disease.

Cravings for high-fat foods and high sugar are usual when one is suffering from low blood sugar. Stable blood sugar levels are necessary for optimum health and to prevent or improve diabetes.

The American Diabetes Association calls lemons and limes "diabetes superfoods," and recommends them for their soluble fiber, their key nutrients, and their contribution to the ever-important low glycemic index. It has been shown that fresh lime or lemon juice can lower the glycemic index of meals up to *thirty percent!*

Lemons & Limes Help Respiratory Disorders Such As Asthma & Bronchitis

Do you suffer from asthma or bronchitis? Scratch the peel of a lime and inhale. It will give you relief from congestion and nausea. The flavonoids in the oil of lemons and limes include kaempferol. Kaempferol is extracted and used in anti-congestive medicines in inhalers, balms, and vaporizers.

A tablespoon of freshly squeezed lemon or lime juice taken an hour before each meal will relieve asthma. Why not try it? You have nothing to lose, and perhaps a whole lot of clear breathing to gain.

Lemons & Limes & Cholesterol

Lemons and limes contain pectin which reduces blood sugar and helps lower harmful LDL cholesterol, while at the same time increasing the levels of the good HDL cholesterol.

Lemons contain as much limonin as they do vitamin C. The phytochemical limonin in lemon juice has also been shown to have LDL cholesterol-lowering effects.

Lab tests by the US Agricultural Research Service (ARS) investigated the process of human liver cells producing less apo B when exposed to limonin. Apo B, a structural protein that is part of the LDL cholesterol molecule, is needed for LDL cholesterol production, transport, and binding. Limonin lowering levels of apo B translated to lower levels of LDL.

Lemons & Limes to the Rescue for Both Constipation & Diarrhea

A digestive system that is not healthy will result in toxins building up and nutrients not being properly absorbed. This condition contributes to bowel discomfort as either constipation or diarrhea.

The simple approach as a preventative to employ for this important attention to your health is once again to drink a glass of room-temperature water with the juice of half a fresh-squeezed lemon or the juice of a whole lime in it every morning.

To cure an existing condition, drink a cup of room-temperature water with fresh squeezed lemon or lime in it with an added pinch of sea salt before each meal. This will activate enzymes and hydrochloric acid (HCL), creating a healthy alkaline environment.

Because lemon or lime juice acts as a cleansing agent and a blood purifier, drinking freshly squeezed lemon or lime juice helps cure constipation by scrubbing off and cleaning the interior walls of the tracts, assisted by the roughage in the lemons and limes. The high level of acids in lemon or lime juice with a pinch of sea salt added is a gentle yet effective purgative. It's an all-natural, healthy process.

Hemorrhoids, too, are cleared up with the lemon or lime treatment. When the citrus fruits have cured constipation and have helped heal ulcers and wounds that may be in the digestive and excretory system, they also have eradicated the root causes of piles.

Diarrhea is the body's way of getting poisons and toxins out of the body. Diarrhea may also indicate a disease process such as ulcerative colitis, dysentery, or irritable bowel syndrome (IBS).

Freshly squeezed lemon or lime juice in a glass of warm water three to five times a day will help eliminate the pathogens that cause diarrhea. The juice also helps prevent dehydration that results from diarrhea. And, of course, daily lemon or lime juice is a great way to prevent these pathogens finding a tolerable environment to multiply in, in the first place.

Lemons & Limes Improve Cystic Fibrosis

Cystic fibrosis patients are advised to consume more foods that decrease mucus production, with lemons and limes at the top of the list.

Cystic fibrosis causes the patient's system to produce too much mucus. This clogs the digestive system and the lungs. Although there is currently no cure for cystic fibrosis, the treatments are intended to help people be successful in managing and improving their symptoms.

Lemon and lime juice is a potentially effective support for the disease treatment regimen, along with the patient's medication and physical therapy.

Lemons & Limes Prevent & Cure Scurvy

As previously mentioned, lemons and limes are historically famous as a cure for scurvy, a disease caused by a deficiency of vitamin C.

The symptoms of scurvy are: frequent infections of cold, coughing, swollen, spongy, bleeding gums, cracked corners of the mouth, cracked lips, and tongue and mouth ulcers, and, without vitamin C, leads to death. Many ships returned to home ports with but skeleton crews until it was understood that the crew needed citrus.

This scourge plagued (and can still plague) miners, too, with their lack of sun and often poor diet. In the present day, people who work in polluted environments such as paint shops, furnaces, cement factories, mines, and the like, need to be attentive to their citrus intake to protect them from scurvy.

Lemons & Limes—Treatment for Cholera & Malaria

Lemon juice and lime juice are blood purifiers. They are therefore the perfect treatment for diseases like cholera and malaria. The potent antibacterial properties in lime and lemon wipe out cholera bacilli in short order.

In villages in West Africa where cholera (triggered by the bacteria, Vibrio cholera) epidemics occur, researchers added lime juice to rice dishes, which proved to protect the people against contracting cholera.

Lemons & Limes Reduce Symptoms of Fibromyalgia, Chronic Fatigue Syndrome & Adrenal Fatigue

Fibromyalgia and chronic fatigue syndrome are frequently discussed together as many of the symptoms are found with both. Also, a notable number of people suffering from one also suffer with the symptoms that are unique to the other.

Fibromyalgia (FM or FMS)

Fibromyalgia is a central nervous system disorder, arising from neurobiological abnormalities which cause physiological pain and can cause cognitive impairments. Fibromyalgia is estimated to affect about four percent of the general population, with women nine times more likely to have it than men.

There are some theories that fibromyalgia may be caused by bacteria or a virus, and, as lemon water alkalizes the body, the proliferation of viruses and harmful bacteria is stopped in its tracks.

Symptoms of fibromyalgia include a painful response to pressure (allodynia) at eighteen tender points, chronic widespread pain, extreme fatigue, joint stiffness, difficulty swallowing, sleep disturbance, muscle spasms, muscle twitching, nerve pain, bowel and bladder abnormalities, tingling, and/or numbness, and possible other issues.

The cognitive complication commonly referred to as "brain fog," or "fibrofog" interferes with concentration, and may cause problems with short and long-term memory, impair speed of performance for tasks and verbal responses, cause challenges with multi-tasking, or shorten attention span.

Chronic Fatigue Syndrome (CFS)

Chronic Fatigue Syndrome (CFS) is a debilitating medical disorder or group of disorders defined as persistent fatigue accompanied by other symptoms.

The disorder is also referred to as chronic fatigue immune dysfunction syndrome (CFIDS), myalgic encephalomyelitis (ME) or post-viral fatigue syndrome (PVFS).

Symptoms of CFS include malaise, poor sleep, widespread joint and muscle pain, muscle weakness, digestive problems, sensitivity to light, sounds and smells, headaches, sore throat, depression, swollen lymph nodes, cardiac and respiratory problems, cognitive difficulties, and chronic, severe, mental and physical exhaustion.

Lemon and lime water can help alleviate the symptoms of fibromyalgia and chronic fatigue in many ways. Following are just a few.

Lemon and lime water help the digestion issues of nausea, heartburn, IBS, constipation and bloating by improving the production of bile, and by detoxing the body.

Lemon and lime water reduces the pain and inflammation of uric acid by dissolving it, and also removes the other acidic wastes from the body.

Adrenal Fatigue

Adrenal fatigue is fatigue that is not relieved by sleep. People suffering from adrenal fatigue may not have any obvious signs of physical illness, yet they live with a pervasive, not-quite-well, tired feeling, often using caffeine and other stimulants to get in motion.

Another great feature of lemon and lime water is that it is a natural energizer, which may help combat chronic fatigue and adrenal fatigue. And, even while it is an energizer, it is also a relaxer, helpful for the stress, anxiety, and depression that the people with FMS, CFS and adrenal fatigue frequently experience.

Lemons & Limes Improve & Heal Ulcers

A stomach ulcer causes severe pain, but it is possible to improve and to cure ulcers. It may seem counterintuitive to add acidic lemon or lime juice to the acid stomach. However, gastric juice in the stomach is an acid four times stronger than the citric acid in lemon juice.

Still, it's advised to "set up" the environment when starting a lemon or lime habit for an ulcer by taking a couple of tablespoons of aloe vera gel before drinking the lemon water to coat the lining of the stomach. Be sure to work in concert with your health care professional.

The stomach produces mucus that lines and protects it from harmful substances. Anything that injures, irritates or thins gastric mucus can initiate ulcers. Introducing the phytochemical limonene to the stomach causes it to produce more mucus.

Researchers at Sao Paolo State University discovered that this protects the stomach from the common cause of ulcers by non-steroidal anti-inflammatories.[5]

The benefits of lemon and lime juice for peptic ulcer, in addition to the great healer, vitamin C, are the limonoid flavonoids—in the form of limonin glucoside and limonene—with their antioxidant, antibiotic and detoxifying processes, which help heal both peptic and oral ulcers.

Lemons & Limes Assist in Healing Autoimmune Disease

Lemon or lime water can assist in healing autoimmune disease in several ways. It significantly aids in digestion and elimination, which helps to prevent toxic build-up in the gut and leaky gut syndrome, as well as other conditions that contribute to the production of allergens in the body. These allergens cause inflammation and disrupt immune system function.

You can help the lemon or lime water do its job by engaging in a thoughtful program of reduced stress, a diet of primarily vegetables and a few fruits, regular exercise, and a commitment to eight hours in bed, fully relaxed. Even if you cannot sleep for eight hours, when you're in bed, completely relaxed, you're getting rest.

Furthermore, you may discover that your body takes a cue from the environment, and you actually begin to sleep more. (Leave your phone by the front door, far from you. Also, shoot your television. Neither the stressors of the EMFs, nor its frequently disturbing content are conducive to sleep, let alone good health.)

Your body knows what it needs, and if you give it lemon or lime water, fresh air, fresh vegetables, and eliminate or greatly reduce processed foods, chemicals, alcohol and environments with toxins (smoking must go!), you'll not only gradually feel fantastic, but you can actually reverse autoimmune disease.

Imagine what life would be like to have your health back!

Lemons & Limes Treat Psoriasis

When the immune system mistakes a normal skin cell for a pathogen and sends out faulty signals that initiate the overproduction of new skin cells, psoriasis is the result.

Unfortunately, psoriasis has been linked to an increased risk of stroke, but research in treating high blood lipid levels appears to lead to improvement of this condition. Drinking lemon and lime water helps normalize high blood lipid levels by making its environment alkaline and hospitable to good health.

In addition, the citric acid in lemon juice applied topically can ameliorate flaking, dryness, and itchiness by helping the skin retain water while encouraging the exfoliation of dead skin cells.

The juice of a lemon contains psoralens, a chemical found in many plants. Psoralens is used in PUVA treatment for psoriasis and eczema as it is highly sensitive to UVA rays.

Ask your dermatologist if the following might be a useful application for your condition: Smooth lemon juice on psoriasis several times a day and then expose to sunlight for a few minutes, gradually increasing the time to sunlight exposure.

Lemons & Limes Heal Infections & Wounds

Lemons and limes are antiseptic. If you increase your intake of lemon or lime for several days when you have an infection or get a wound, it will speed up the healing process. The body knows how to heal itself, and when it's damaged it uses the body's resources of vitamin C to send to the infection or wound to heal it and to initiate collagen formation.

It's suggested to drink the juice of two or three lemons or four or five limes daily, in room temperature water while the infection or wound heals.

Lemons & Limes Make Smooth Electrical Transmissions for the Brain & Nervous System

Lemons and limes are high in potassium, which is an important mineral that works together with sodium to produce smooth electrical transmissions in the nervous system and the brain.

"Brain fog," forgetfulness, anxiety, and depression are often caused by low levels of potassium in the blood. Potassium provides the nervous system the signals necessary for steady, healthy functioning.

When electrodes are hooked up to lemons, they act as a battery, running electrical current. This is a graphic representation of their electrical conductivity, so it's easy to see that this electrical conductivity makes the brain and nervous system run smoothly. Lemons and limes can run a clock, and they can keep you ticking, too!

Lemons & Limes Help Make Baby

Cervical fluid, which is naturally acidic, is influenced by the body's pH levels. Therefore drinking lemon water is helpful to assist in its alkalinity when pregnant or intending to become pregnant. This alkaline environment is necessary to protect sperm and egg cells, and the precious DNA. Once again, the antioxidants in lemons and limes help protect cells from free radical damage, which is of paramount importance in the delicate uterine garden.

Lemons & Limes Contribute to Weight Loss

Getting into a daily habit of having fresh squeezed lemon or lime juice significantly contributes to a healthy weight-loss program (which, of course, needs also to include a well-balanced diet and exercise).

A glass of room-temperature water with fresh squeezed lemon or lime juice is not only a great weight reducer, but it boosts your whole system with its antioxidant and other health-stimulating components.

Lemon water stimulates digestive enzymes and hydrochloric acid (HCL). This provides at least two beneficial processes: your stomach can better digest foods, and your system will increase its utilization of fats. This, in turn, results in long-term weight loss.

Don't forget that adequate water is an extremely important component of weight loss. It hydrates you so your body can flush out all the waste and excess weight it's trying to release, and water also contributes to feeling full. Oh boy—win-win! Have two glasses of lemon or lime juice a day to enjoy the many benefits of gradual weight loss—bright skin, easier movement, more energy, joyful mood, deep sleep—and the list goes on.

The citric acid in lemons and limes burns fat, plus it's all natural. And affordable! No need to buy into complicated, expensive and often health-compromising weight-loss programs. Just appreciate Mother Nature's perfect weight-loss remedy in neat, entirely biodegradable, brightly-colored packages in the form of lemons and limes, and the excess-weight will burn off, in a gradual and healthy manner.

Insulin and hormone production stores fat. We crave high sugar and high-fat foods when experiencing low blood sugar. Lemon and lime water nourishes the liver's enzymes and stimulates it. This increases your body's ability to clear out the toxins, further contributing to weight loss.

And, yes, there's more! Lemon or lime juice aids in weight loss, because, (as noted under *Lemons & Limes & Diabetes*, above) its high vitamin content helps to stabilize blood sugar levels by regulating sugar absorption and regulating your metabolism. Your body needs stable blood sugar for weight loss, and it needs stable blood sugar to maintain its best weight once you get to your goal.

The chemistry of lemon and lime juice makes water more bioavailable. And, last but certainly not least in this impressive list of healthy weight loss, these cheerful citrus give the water a bright, refreshing and interesting taste, contributing to reducing the psychological (in addition to the physiological) aspect of feeling hungry. In the end, taste can be the most critical factor.

Lemons & Limes Battle Colds, Influenza, Fever & Sore Throat

First of all, let's do our best to avoid suffering with a cold, influenza, fever or a sore throat in the first place. Your primary line of defense in this effort is vitamin C, found in larger quantities-per-volume in lemons and limes than in almost any other fruit or vegetable. Daily intake of lime or lemon juice will ward off opportunistic, nasty bugs.

If you get a sore throat, gargling with straight lemon or lime juice is very beneficial. If the straight juice is too much for you, you can cut it with water, but pure juice is more effective. The antibacterial property of lemons and limes makes them an excellent means to assist in getting rid of throat infections and will help relieve the symptoms of tonsillitis as well.

If you're running a fever, lemon or lime juice helps to break the fever by increasing perspiration, while the ascorbic acid contributes to reducing coughing and phlegm.

You can make yourself a glass of warm lemonade or limeade to sip on, and it will not only soothe your throat, but all of the health benefits of the vitamins, flavonoids, and enzymes in the lemon and lime will contribute to your rapid healing from your sore throat, fever, cold or flu.

The Linus Pauling Institute states that the high content of vitamin C in lemons and limes can reduce the duration of a cold by as much as 14 percent.[6]

Lemons & Limes for Strong Teeth & Healthy Eyes

When it comes to caring for your miraculous, amazing eyes, it's vitamin C in lemons and limes to the rescue yet again. Because of vitamin C's antioxidant properties, your eyes are protected from macular degeneration, cataracts and other eye problems attributed to aging, and the lemon and lime flavonoids help protect your precious eyes from infections.

And here's some information about lemons and limes for your gums, mouth, and teeth. Gums really take a beating, and when they weaken, you can start to lose your teeth as well. The first and biggest problem for gums is generally a vitamin C deficiency, which is seen to a dramatic degree with people who have scurvy, with bleeding, spongy gums.

Without adequate vitamin C, there is unhealthy microbial growth. Mouth ulcers and wounds may also develop. Lemon and lime juice is your mouth's friend. The vitamin C shores up overall health, the potassium and flavonoids heal the wounds and ulcers, and the flavonoids stop the microbial growth.

Lemons and limes improve halitosis. Lemon and lime juice makes an excellent mouthwash, removes plaque, and whitens teeth, as lemons and limes can serve as a bleaching agent. Again, be sure to rinse with water, as the acidic content of lemons and limes may damage tooth enamel.

If you are currently in mouth pain, a glass of room temperature water with a pinch of sea salt and half a fresh lemon or a whole lime squeezed into it will begin to relieve your pain and reduce swelling. Lemon and lime juice will relieve gingivitis, tongue inflammation, and stomatitis.

Rub the white inside of the rind—also known as the albedo—on the gums to assist in the healing process.

You can massage fresh-squeezed lemon juice on a toothache and it will reduce the pain. If there's bleeding, it will staunch the blood until you get to your dentist.

Caution: DO NOT put off going to the dentist if you have a toothache or other dental problem.

Lemons & Limes Stop Heartburn

As mentioned before, drink the juice of ½ lemon or a whole lime in a glass of room-temperature water to relieve, and probably dispel, heartburn.

Lemons & Limes Improve Allergies

Allergies make people sneeze, feel congested, clogged with mucus, and itchy. Allergies wear people down, making them feel tired and irritable. Allergens disrupt the immune system with inflammation.

Lemon or lime water prevents toxic buildup in the system that causes the production of allergens instigating this inflammation and congestion. It boosts the immune system, thinning mucus and unclogging the sinuses.

Lemons & Limes Reduce Soreness After a Workout

Lemons and limes alkalize the body, so drinking the juice regularly reduces the buildup of lactic acid, which will help alleviate the pain caused by the tiny tears that occur in the muscles during a workout. Drinking a liter of lemon water with a bit of sea salt in it after a workout will help replenish your electrolytes.

Lemons & Limes Make Hair Beautiful

Lemon and lime juice removes product buildup in hair, and, as lemons are a gentle bleaching agent, it's a perfect natural highlighter. Because it's natural, there is not the risk of allergic reaction that people often have to hair dyes.

Just applying lemon juice to the hair gives it a beautiful shine. But lemon and lime juice can take care of serious concerns with hair, too. Applying the juice to the scalp will treat dandruff, and has even been reported to return the growth of hair to bald spots.

Lemons & Limes & Radiant Skin

If you really want to glow on the outside, you have to take care of the inside first. Lemon and lime on a daily basis will give you beautiful skin if you're not eating junk food and are getting adequate sleep and exercise.

Lemon and lime juice is a natural antiseptic, and as such can help cure skin problems. In addition to drinking the juice, apply it topically to a sting or to sunburn to relieve the pain and help your skin heal. You can also apply lemon or lime juice to acne, eczema or burn scars for a healing result and to diminish scarring.

Lemons and limes will protect your skin from infections and cure rashes and bruises. They will make your skin look young, minimize wrinkles and lines and do away with blackheads, age spots, and skin tags. Lemon juice also relieves itchy skin and chilblains.

If you have dry skin, or a dry skin patch, rub the peel of a lemon or lime on the dry or scaly skin, and be prepared to be amazed at the restored moisture and softness. All of these benefits are due to vitamin C and to the flavonoid's antioxidant, antibiotic and disinfectant processes.

Lemon juice is a good and natural bleach for skin, too. It reduces the pigment melanin. There is no risk of chemical allergic reactions as is common with chemical bleaches.

Use the entire fruit—the pulp segments, albedo, and rind. Each of the three components adds something different to the healing mix.

Rub the albedo, the white part, on skin problems. Then abrade the outside of the peel with a knife or grater so that the oils are accessible, and rub that on your skin as well. Be sure the fruit has been well-scrubbed before you cut into it so that any possible pesticides or wax coating is removed.

Add lemon or lime juice and their oil to your bath and give all of your skin the advantages of their wonderful benefits. In addition, lemons and limes do away with body odor.

It's best to soak the fruits in a sink of tepid water (neither hot nor cold) and a spoonful of sea salt for ten minutes when you bring them home to rid them of any pesticides or microorganisms, so that you can use the skins without concern of coming in contact with substances that are counterproductive to your goal of radiant, beautiful skin.

CHAPTER HIGH POINTS:

1. Lemons and limes have an atomic structure similar to the human body's hydrochloric acid, bile, and saliva, which assists in the digestion of food.

2. The citric acid in lemons and limes is the number one carrier of biochemicals in the body.

3. Fresh lemon or lime juice can be used by the liver for enzyme production *more effectively than any other food*.

4. Lemons and limes have a high potassium content which:

   a. has been scientifically linked to stabilizing blood pressure, providing the nervous system with clear pathways to send steady signals to the heart.

   b. prevents nausea and dizziness because of the regulated blood pressure, and reduces depression and emotional stress.

   c. works in concert with sodium to produce smooth electrical transmissions in the nervous system and the brain.

5. Lemons and limes contain the disease-fighting compounds known as flavonoids, which are extremely bioavailable. Flavonoids have antioxidant, anticancer, antiallergic, anti-inflammatory, anti-microbial and anti-diarrheal properties. They modify viruses and carcinogens and can even induce cancer cell death.

The flavonoid naringenin, in the skins of lemons and limes, is a rich antioxidant, free radical scavenger, and anti-inflammatory. Naringenin minimizes cancer development, promotes carbohydrate metabolism and modulates the immune system. It helps prevent damage to DNA and even *repairs* DNA.

6. The American Diabetes Association calls lemons and limes "diabetes superfoods," for their soluble fiber, their key nutrients, and their contribution to lowering blood sugars. Fresh lime or lemon juice can lower the glycemic index of meals up to *thirty percent!*

7. Vitamin C is found in larger quantities-per-volume in lemons and limes than in almost any other fruit or vegetable.

8. Plus a plethora of other amazing contributions to health, happiness, and beauty.

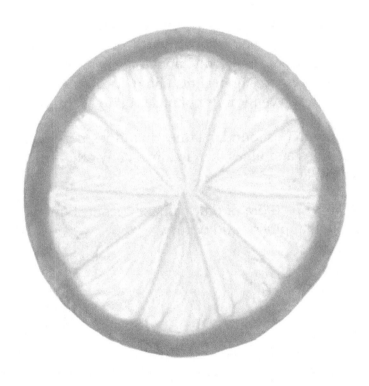

Chapter 4:
Uses of Lemons & Limes in Cooking

"Food, like your money,
should be working for you!"

Rita Dettrea Beckford, M.D.

Lemons and limes are used throughout the world in a variety of foods entirely too numerous to list. But here you'll find a few uses that you can put into practice, so that, along with their medicinal value, you'll get to enjoy their delightful, tantalizing flavors.

As mentioned before, lemon pickle is a common condiment on many tables. If you've never tried it, you can get a jar from your local Asian, East Indian or health food store to complement your meals and to use as a digestive aid.

Lemon and lime juice and zest from the rind are components of many foods and drinks. They are used as a marinade for cooking, in soft drinks and cocktails. The grated zest of lemon and lime rind adds flavor, fiber and health benefits to rice dishes, desserts, cooking, baking, and drinks. There are zesters available, or you can also use a vegetable peeler to peel off just the thin, colorful layer of the peel for your zest.

Lemon juice is also a preservative for foods that oxidize and turn brown after being sliced, such as avocados, bananas, peaches, apricots, and apples. The acid in lemon juice disrupts the process of the enzymes that cause browning and degradation.

Lemon or lime juice drizzled over other fruits, over grilled vegetables and other foods enhances their flavors. And, of course, a lemon or lime slice or curl of rind is used as a decorative garnish on many dishes, desserts and drinks to add interest and color.

Whole, dried lemons are a part of Moroccan, Middle Eastern, and East Indian cuisine. A tea is made from the leaves of the lemon tree, and the leaves are also used in cooking.

Fresh-squeezed lemon or lime juice with crushed garlic cloves and extra virgin olive oil makes a delightful, refreshing salad dressing, while lime juice squeezed onto an avocado is a meal all by itself. Lemon or lime wedges with a meal add *zing!* and can replace salt.

The alluring aroma and tang of lime flavor is the favorite of many people. Lime is found all around the globe in snacks, jams, jellies, candies, sorbets, sherbet, as a marinade, and in refreshing drinks. Don't forget the Key lime pie!

Lemon Pickle Recipe

Ingredients, etc:

8 unwaxed or organic lemons

4-5 tbsp sea salt

4-5 tbsp red chili powder - to taste

2 tbsp fenugreek seeds/or 1 tsp roasted and ground fenugreek for the seasoning

2 tbsp peanut oil

½ tsp mustard seeds

Other:

1 lb capacity wide mouth glass/porcelain jar with a tight-fitting lid

Parchment paper - as a barrier between the salt in the pickle and the metal lid. Otherwise, use a piece of muslin or cotton

Glass, porcelain, or stainless steel mixing bowl

Long spoon

Preparation:

Wash the glass or porcelain jar well with hot water and soap and let air dry completely.

All the working surfaces and utensils need to be completely clean and dry.

Wash the lemons and pat them dry with a fresh, clean kitchen towel.

Quarter the lemons.

There must be NO MOISTURE in the jar or on the lemons.

Add ½ tsp of salt to the bottom of the lemon pickle jar.

Add the lemon pieces and salt in alternating layers until all lemon pieces are covered in salt including the top layer.

Cut out the parchment paper slightly bigger than the lid, line it in the lid and secure tightly.

Let the jar of lemons sit for 7-10 days in a cool, dry spot.

Shake or stir with a long dry spoon once a day.

Add Spices:

After 7-10 days, in a small pan dry roast the fenugreek seeds on low heat until fragrant and golden brown. (Do not over-roast or they will become bitter.)

When cool, grind the seeds to a fine powder.

In a clean, dry glass bowl mix red chili powder and the roasted, ground fenugreek. Empty the jar of preserved lemons into the bowl of spice and mix well with a dry spoon.

Heat oil in a small pan. Add mustard seeds and cook until they sputter.

As the sputtering stops, take the mustard seeds off the stove and cool.

Add mustard seeds to the lemon pickle, and stir.

Carefully return the pickle back to the jar.

Seal the parchment paper lined lid tightly again. Let the pickle soak all the spices for at least two days before using.

Never mix or handle the pickle with your hand, it will spoil the pickle.

You don't need to refrigerate the lemon pickle as it keeps for a long time if properly stored.

YUM!

CHAPTER HIGH POINTS:

1. Lemon and lime pickle is a common condiment that is also a digestive aid.

2. Lemons and limes add a piquant flavor to dishes ranging from beverages to the main dish, to desserts.

3. Fruits and vegetables that rapidly oxidize are preserved by drizzling lemon or lime juice over them, thereby extending their usefulness.

4. The aroma of lemon and lime adds a subtle dimension to any culinary application.

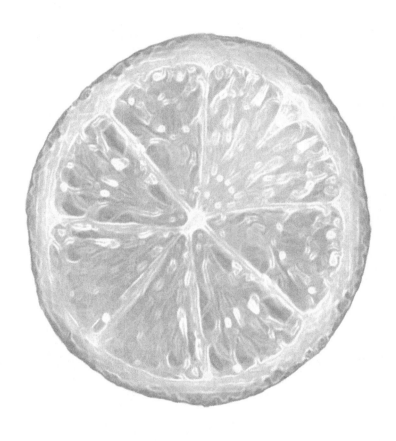

Chapter 5:
Miscellaneous Lemon & Lime Uses & Remedies

> *"The doctor of the future will no longer treat the human frame with drugs, but rather will cure and prevent disease with nutrition."*
> Thomas Edison

One could probably compile several volumes of all the ways in which lemons and limes have been used by the human family throughout time and cultures. The following information recounts just a few of the numerous applications where lemon or lime has been discovered to be of benefit.

Lemon is a nontoxic insecticide and repels mosquitoes. Think "citronella." As an insect repellent, add

15-25 drops of lemon oil to a cup of water in a spray bottle.

Do you have a painful corn? Put a slice of lemon on it, and wrap it overnight. You will be relieved of the pain, and the corn will start to heal. Or you can use lemon essential oil as well on the corn. Dab it on with a cotton swab, but avoid letting the undiluted oil touch un-callused skin.

Lemon oil reduces pain. Mix a few drops with a couple of teaspoons of jojoba oil and gently massage an inflamed area. Use this same mixture to rub on spider veins or varicose veins daily to reduce their appearance.

Lemon juice on a cotton swab placed in the nose will stop a nose bleed.

A hemorrhage can be checked by taking lemon juice because of its styptic and antiseptic properties. Drink this lemon water *ice cold*—as an exception to the directions everywhere else in the book—the cold will assist in staunching the hemorrhage.

Cool lemonade or limeade contributes to being cool and calm, and, although probably not as effective as lemon juice at body temperature in some ways, its cooling influence when you're hot and sweaty is very important and thus effective in other ways.

As an aromatic, lemon oil smells fresh and clean and has been shown to help concentration. Place a few drops of the essential lemon oil in an aromatic warmer when studying for an exam, or any other activity requiring your undivided attention.

Hot feet: Our feet take a lot of abuse and rarely get the attention they deserve. So take some time to give your feet a bit of love.

If the soles of your feet are burning, rub a slice of lemon or lime over the bottom of your feet. This will cool them, relieve the pain, and it will also pull toxins that gather in the bottom of your feet out through their pores.

You can take it "one step further" and soak your tired feet in a tub of warm water with lemon *or* lime or lemon *and* lime in it. Enjoy the lovely, relaxing sensation and the delicate aromatic of the lemon or lime, which is also relaxing. The astringent, antiseptic nature of lemon and lime will remove tension and alleviate exhaustion. Afterward, you'll sleep like a baby (if you don't fall asleep right there!).

Dried lemon and lime has been used for many applications. Try this: peel a lemon or lime, let the peelings dry in sunlight, then grind them up and keep on hand if you are prone to headaches. Apply this powder to you head before taking a bath—it will relieve your headache and cool your body.

Bind a slice of lemon or lime over a whitlow, which is an abscess in the soft tissue near a fingernail or toenail, and it will bring the discharge to the surface where you can clean it out. With lemon or lime applied, it will quickly heal.

Lime oil is extracted from the lime's peel and used in not only edible products but also in body oils, oils for the hair, toothpaste, soap, mouthwashes, deodorants, disinfectants, and cosmetics.

Lemon oil is common in cleaning products. You can make your own. It's not only the clean scent of lemons and limes that we like in our cleaning products, but the oil also works as a solvent that dissolves dirt, grime, fingerprints, and other substances that find their way onto our furniture. Lemon oil reconditions wood, which you'll notice when the wood appears to drink it up and shine beautifully.

Lemon, with its antibiotic chemistry, makes a great cleaner, and you'll notice that its bleaching attribute removes stains. Add baking soda for an abrasive and as an additional neutralizing cleaner. You can take half a lemon, dip it in salt or baking powder and make all your copper-bottomed pans, or anything else you have that's copper, shine like new because the acid in the lemon dissolves the tarnish.

The juice of lemons and limes removes grease, deodorizes and disinfects in the kitchen and the bathroom. It removes stains from plastic when combined with baking soda.

Citron, although the fruit is essentially inedible, keeps moths out of clothing and linens.

CHAPTER HIGH POINTS:

1. Lemon is a non-toxic insecticide.

2. Lemon and lime oil reduces pain.

3. Lemon oil and lemon juice are astringent, antiseptic and styptic. It can staunch the flow of blood of everything from a nose bleed to an internal hemorrhage.

4. The aroma of lemon oil helps concentration.

5. Feet and heads love lemon and lime. Various applications relieve exhaustion and pain.

6. As a cleaner, lemon juice or oil removes stains and grease, conditions wood, and deodorizes and disinfects the whole house.

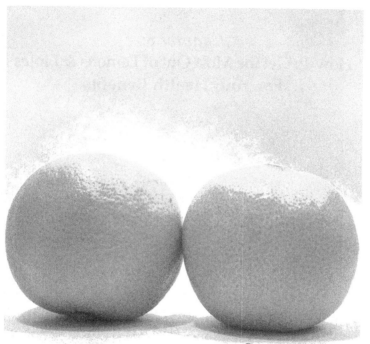

Sweet Limes

Chapter 6:
How To Get the Most Out of Lemons & Limes
For Your Health Benefits

*"Any food that requires the use
of chemical substances should
in no way be considered a food."*
John H. Tobe

The best way to get the most out of your daily fresh squeezed lemon or lime is with spring water, at between room and body temperature. The lemon or lime also needs to be at room temperature. This is because the enzymes and nutritional value are most readily used up by your body when the fruit is at room temperature.

If you drink your lemon or lime in hot water, the hot water destroys enzymes and other nutrients, and if ice cold, your body has to work hard to heat the water up—since all the digestive processes in the body are chemical reactions that generate heat—before it can absorb the nutritional components. Because of this, the enzymes and other components are not fully used, as the body is expending its energy in heating the components, rather than assimilating the nutritional value.

If you're taking the fruit from the refrigerator, let it stand in warm water for a while to warm up. Another way of getting the most juice that a lemon or lime has to offer is to roll it under hand on the counter. This loosens the segments from the pulp. You'll notice a lot more juice with this method when hand-squeezing the fruit.

Be sure to scrub the fruit before cutting it to assure that there are no pesticides, organisms, or the nearly undetectable wax on the skins. It's best to put all your fruit and vegetables in a sink of room temperature water with a tablespoon of sea salt and let them soak for about ten minutes when you first get them home to disarm pesticides and organisms.

There are, of course, lemon/lime squeezers, which are smaller than ones for oranges. However, I've discovered making an "X" through the segments in the half lemon or lime that is warm and that I've rolled under hand works very well with my orange squeezer, which otherwise is perfect as it's attached to a glass container, and rinsing all the goodie from the top washes right down into the container. This perfectly fills the cup I pour it into.

Drink your lemon or lime water straight, without any sweetener, and drink it right down. *Don't wait!* Enzymes are short-lived, so to get their goodness they need to go in your system right away.

If you have a juicer, you can throw the whole fruit in. But another possible advantage of hand juicing is that you're left with the albedo—the white part—and the rind.

You can cut the rind in half and flatten it, then rub both sides on your skin for clearing the complexion, brightening the skin, smoothing rough patches on elbows or feet, fading spots, or reducing wrinkles. You can also put the rinds in your bath for their aromatic, skin smoothing, skin healing, relaxing benefits.

It is generally recommended to drink your lemon or lime water upon awakening, an hour before any other beverage and before eating. Ultimately, this is an excellent goal. But this habit is one that you're acquiring for a lifetime, and drinking a tall glass of unsweetened lemon or lime juice right when you wake up may not seem like much fun at first. So do it in a way that you know you'll continue. It took me two weeks to get to the point of doing it first thing in the morning every morning.

Another thing you'll notice as you become more pH balanced if lemon is very bitter to you—it becomes less and less bitter as you daily drink your lemon or lime juice. In other words, when you are less acidic, the lemon or lime tastes less acidic. So if lemon is difficult for you to take, remember, this means you really need it, and it will get better over time.

Also, keep in mind that the fantastic components of these citrus are more effective in a body that has fasted overnight.

It's recommended that the goal for people who weigh under 150 pounds is one lemon (or equivalent volume of lime) every day, and for people who weigh over 150 pounds two lemons (or equivalent volume of lime) a day. Clearly, this is a rough guideline. Start out slow but steady, and over time you will discover how much lemon and/or lime water your body requires to achieve maximum results.

Five Times More Bioavailable

Don't forget that the wonderful flavonoid, limonene, and the highest concentration of vitamin C, is found in the albedo—the pith of the lemon or lime. You may want to eat this from time to time, as well as make a zest from the rinds to put in or on your cooking or desserts.

As previously mentioned, lemon and lime make the other nutrients in what you consume more bioavailable—*as much as five times more available!*

Freezing

You can also juice lemons and limes and freeze the juice in ice cube trays, then store, tightly sealed, in the freezer. This is useful for people who cannot always get lemons or limes, or to pop a couple into a glass of water for a refreshing drink.

Just keep in mind that although the vitamins and minerals remain effective, the enzymes, phytonutrients, and biophotons probably do not after the juice has been exposed to air and frozen.

Shopping Tips

Organic fruits are best. But, once again, any fresh lemon or lime is better than none.

When you buy lemons and limes, look at the stem end, that is, the end where you can see the fruit hung from the tree. You will see lines that radiate out from the center. This is called a calyx. The more lines the calyx has, the more minerals the fruit has, and this is good.

Buy thin-skinned and finely grained lemons that are rather heavier for their size, as they have more flesh and more juice. Choose lemons that are completely yellow, they are more ripe than ones that have green tinges. Over-ripe lemons are dull in color, have hard or soft patches on them, and their skin is less smooth.

Choose limes that are deep green, unless you're getting one of the yellow lime varieties. Again, look for a smooth, glossy, firm skin. Even green limes eventually turn yellow. However, they are at the height of their ripeness and flavor when they are the most intense green color.

Lemons and limes will keep for a long time in the refrigerator, but they lose their flavor over time. Outside of the refrigerator, they will stay fresh for one to perhaps two weeks, if kept out of sunlight. If you want them to ripen, place them in the sunlight.

Store lemon and lime zest in a sealed glass container in the refrigerator.

Other Considerations

Be sure to have the other half of your lemon or lime in the evening. It's believed that a cut lemon or lime loses its efficacy, so keep it face down, preferably against glass in a glass jar with the lid on, to keep it as "sealed" as possible.

If, at first, a whole lemon a day is too much (not as likely with limes, as they are smaller) then have the other half the next morning. Lemons and limes oxidize slowly, and their goodness, if kept enclosed, should last a day.

To get the most antioxidants, carefully choose fully ripe lemons and limes. Antioxidant levels increase as fruit ripens, according to research done at the University of Innsbruck in Austria.[7]

Researchers identified polar nonflourescing chlorophyll catabolytes (NCCs) in fruit as they become very ripe. NCCs are unusually powerful antioxidants that protect the fruit when it is fully ripe. These NCCs have the same protective effect when we eat them.[8]

Testimonials

Following are some testimonials about the miraculous efficacy of fresh lemons and limes. Let me share a story of one of my friends, followed by some others:

The friend of one of my friends in a class I was taking had a terrible infection with his big toe. It became so serious that they were talking about amputation if it didn't begin to heal.

She showed me a picture of his toe that she had on her phone. I was flabbergasted—the toe looked like it was about to explode, was dark, angry red and nearly as big as his foot! I told her that his pH was very acidic and that he had nothing to lose by drinking the juice of a lot of fresh lemons.

As much as I believe in the power of alkalizing the body, even I was amazed when my friend came into class the very next week and said that her friend's toe had almost completely healed! His doctor was also amazed.

Here are some more experiences people have shared with me regarding getting on the lemon and lime habit:

"I am 74 years young. Within a day of doing lemons I noticed my stomach didn't feel as bloated as it had been. Around day three I noticed my sugar cravings were less. I also feel it's helped with my blood pressure. My blood pressure has been very high, often over 200 on the top. The blood pressure pills my doctor prescribed didn't bring it down hardly at all. This was with being on several different blood pressure medications, all of which gave me terrible side effects. I finally told the doctor that I wanted to try alternative methods and he agreed.

"I started drinking lemon or lime water twice a day, night and morning as suggested. Sometimes when I feel I need it, I take an extra dose. I just got back from my monthly visit with my blood pressure doctor, and after only three weeks drinking lemon water, my blood pressure is down to an average of 178—from over 200! The doc took it three times to make sure. He told me to keep doing what I was doing.

"I also take medication for water retention and often, even if I take it in the morning, it doesn't seem to take effect until bedtime which means I'm up all night going to the bathroom. Since starting lemons I sleep better through the night, getting up only once or maybe twice instead of three and four times. I plan on continuing my lemon and healthier eating regime and am optimistic that my blood pressure will continue to drop.

"I have also noticed my skin feels smoother. My family and friends have commented on my youthful appearance!"

Gayla J.

(Editor's note: A month later Gayla's blood pressure dropped another 12 points. Her doctor said again, "Keep doing what you're doing!")

———

"After a mere four days of ½ of a lemon sometime during the day, a pencil lead-sized skin-tag-or-whatever-it-was that had appeared on my forehead six months previous, that I had scrubbed and scrubbed hoping to remove, but it only got bigger, had just simply *disappeared*! Another slightly larger something that I'd had on my cheek for years was all but gone in ten days, and then, soon after, vanished.

"Many other positive results have been ongoing. I dropped ten pounds in five weeks. I'm a convert!"

Joann N.

"I've had a really ugly infestation of Seborrhoeic Keratosis, which is a fungus. I tried everything, and spent a lot of money on products that made no difference whatsoever. These spots weren't just icky looking, they caught on clothing and sometimes tore and bled, and it smelled. Altogether horrible.

"I stopped all these things I was trying and started to 'do' the lemon/lime routine. In addition to drinking the juice of a lemon or lime in the morning and evening, I'd rub the inside and the outside of the lemon or lime skin on all these ugly brown growths.

"I couldn't believe it when the bad smell went away the second day, and all the tiny growths, *poof!* disappeared in 4 days. Now, three weeks later, the big ones are almost flat and are rapidly fading.

"I've been fighting this fungus for over five years, but with lemons and limes, miraculously, in less than a month, it's almost gone.

"And there's all these other unanticipated benefits. I'm sleeping soundly, which is something new, and I wake up wide awake and ready to jump out of bed. I haven't felt like this since I was a kid.

"Hooray for lemons and limes!!!"

Anonymous

"My friend, who is a friend of Dr. Ayne, nagged me so much about 'doing the lemon/lime thing' that I started doing it. I didn't have any particular thing in mind to improve. My friend just said it would make me healthier. I didn't exactly believe it, but, I figured, nothing to lose.

"Surprise! After a few days, I noticed that it felt like I was breathing so much air! I didn't even know my sinuses were sort of swollen. It's fantastic, all this air.

"And then there was another weird thing. I crave chocolate. I don't have it every day, but I'm pretty sure I think about it every day. Yesterday I walked by a rack of candy bars in the grocery store and realized that I hadn't even thought of chocolate in several days. Like I say, weird."

K.'s Friend

———————

And this from your author:

I know about pH balance. After all, I wrote the book, *Save Your Life with the Power of pH Balance.* I knew lemons and limes were good for you. But I didn't get into the serious routine of lemon or lime every day until I started to do the research on this book.

As an author, I have my eyes on a computer screen many hours a day. I've noticed, over the last few months, that, when I leave the computer to go for a walk, it takes ten or fifteen minutes for my eyes to adjust to clearly see at-distance trees. I was sad to see my eyes faltering.

But about a week after starting my lemon/lime routine, I was stunned when I went out for my walk and noticed there was something dramatically different. The trees seemed, at first, to be very bright, and then I realized that I was seeing things—both near and far—extremely clearly!

Then I had a second wonderful experience. When I'm hard at work with my glasses on, if I look out the window, I noticed a few months ago, the trees had the same clarity as my computer screen. It had previously been that I'd have to take my glasses off for the trees to be clear. So this was another confirmation that my at-distance vision was faltering.

A couple of days ago, I paused, looked out the window, and noticed the trees were very blurry. Then I took off my glasses and the trees became clear. In less than two weeks on the lemon/lime regime, my eyes have improved flat out amazingly.

It seems to me that just this one potential improvement would excite anyone to get on the lemon/lime train.

Just Do It!

So, just do it! *A minimum* of one-half of a fresh-squeezed lemon or a whole lime—Every. Single. Day. No If. No And. No But.

Dramatic results come with faithful daily intake, and even more so when you drink your lemon or lime water first thing in the morning. And even *more* more so when you have it both morning and evening.

Healing Crisis

However, do be prepared for a possible "healing crisis." It knocked me for a loop after about eight days. I hurt everywhere and felt awful. At first, I couldn't figure it out. Then I realized that the lemon and lime were clearing out deep-seated toxins and contaminants. My body was gung-ho for the spring cleaning.

Fortunately, I was aware of the healing crisis (discussed at some length in *Save Your Life with the Power of pH Balance*) and I was ready to see it through.

As my diet and life-style are already healthy, my healing crisis passed in a couple days. A healing crisis is something that can vary considerably—you may not experience it at all. But if you do, ride it out.

You won't believe how energized, cleared, and emotionally bright you'll feel when you come through to the other side.

Do you have a lemon/lime testimonial you'd like to share with others? If so, you may send it along:

Blythe@BlytheAyne.com

CHAPTER HIGH POINTS:

1. Have your daily fresh squeezed lemon or lime at room temperature, ideally with spring or ionized water, also at room temperature. But if you only have tap water, have the juice with tap water.

2. Scrub the fruit before cutting it to assure that there are no pesticides, organisms, or the nearly undetectable wax on the skins.

3. First roll the lemon or lime under hand on the counter, loosening the segments from the pulp.

4. Put your fruit and vegetables in a sink of room temperature water with a tablespoon of sea salt and let them soak for ten minutes to disarm pesticides and organisms.

5. Cut the juiced rind in half and flatten, then rub both sides on your skin for clearing the complexion, brightening the skin, smoothing rough patches on elbows or feet, fading spots, or reducing wrinkles. Then put the rinds in the bath for aromatic, skin smoothing, skin healing, relaxing benefits.

6. The goal is to drink your lemon or lime water upon awakening, an hour before any other beverage and before eating.

7. Ultimate goal: If you weigh under 150 pounds, one lemon (or equivalent amount of lime) every

day. If you weigh over 150 pounds, two lemons (or equivalent amount of lime) a day.

8. Lemons and limes make the other nutrients in what you consume up to five times more bioavailable.

9. Look for thin-skinned, heavy (contains more juice) fruit, with several mineral-content lines radiating from the calyx.

10. Buy organic when you can.

11. Antioxidant levels increase as fruit ripens. Polar nonflourescing chlorophyll catabolytes (NCCs) in fruit are unusually powerful antioxidants that protect the fruit when it is fully ripe and have the same protective effect on you when you eat them.

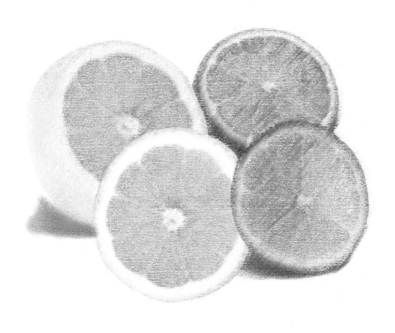

Chapter 7:
What's in These Lovely Fruits to Make Them So Potent?

"Bear in mind that some substances that are alkaline outside the body are acidic to the body, meaning that they leave an acid residue in the tissues, just as many substances that are acidic outside the body, like lemons, are alkaline and healing in the body and contribute to the body's critical alkaline reserve."

Natalia Rose,
Detox for Women: An All New Approach

We see that lemons and limes have high nutrient value. They are full of antioxidants to fight free radical damage. They contain enzymes, biophotons, and phytonutrients, that, although short-lived after the fruit is cut, are nothing short of miraculous components, curing diseases and manifesting health.

They contain a complex of B vitamins, vitamin C, iron, potassium, omega-3 fatty acids, omega-6 fatty acids, and a host of other vitamins and minerals, as noted below, and they are also a very good source of dietary fiber.

What's the Difference Between Lemons and Limes?

Lemons are more tart than limes. Limes have a higher percentage of citric acid. Both juices are used to add strong, mouth-watering flavor and aroma to a meal. Both juices have preservative qualities.

There is the obvious color difference, although there are wonderful yellow limes, and lemons are green before they turn yellow. Generally speaking, limes are smaller than lemons.

Below is the list of the components of lemons and limes. As you can see, lemons have more vitamin C and a bit more potassium per equal measure, and limes have more vitamin A and calcium per equal measure. Other components are quite similar or with negligible differences.

Nutrition of Fresh Lemons
Per 100 Grams & Percent of Daily Values:

Species:	*Citrus x limon*	
Taste:	Sour	
Carbohydrates	9.32 g	(3%)
Sugars	3.50 g	
Dietary fiber	3 g	(11%)
Protein	1.10 g	
Vitamins and Minerals:		
Vitamin A, Retinol	22.0 IU	(<1%)
B Vitamins in lemons:		
Thiamine, vitamin B_1	0.04 mg	(3%)
Riboflavin, vitamin B_2	0.02 mg	(2%)
Niacin, vitamin B_3	0.10 mg	(1%)
Pantothenic acid, vitamin B_5	0.19 mg	(2%)
Vitamin B_6	.010 mg	(4%)
Folate, vitamin B_9	11 mcg	(3%)
Vitamin C	53 mg	(88%)
Calcium	25 mg	(3%)
Choline	5.10 mg	
Copper	0.08 mg	(2%)
Vitamin E (Alpha Tocopherol)	0.22 mg	(0%)
Electrolytes		
Flavonoids		
Iron	0.60 mg	(5%)
Vitamin K	0.00 mcg	(0%)
Magnesium	8 mg	(2%)
Manganese	trace	
Phosphorus	16 mg	(2%)
Potassium	138 mg	(3%)
Selenium	0.40 mcg	(1%)
Zinc	0.06 mg	(1%)
Total Omega-3 fatty acids	26 mg	
Total Omega-6 fatty acids	63 mg	
Calories	29	(2%)

Nutrition of Fresh Limes
Per 100 Grams & Percent of Daily Values:

Species:	*Citrus x latifolia*	
Taste:	Bitter/Sweet	
Carbohydrates	11 g	(4%)
Sugars	2 g	
Dietary fiber	3 g	(11%)
Protein	.7 g	(1%)
Vitamins and Minerals:		
Vitamin A, Retinol	50.0 IU	(1%)
B Vitamins in limes:		
Thiamine, vitamin B_1	0.03 mg	(2%)
Riboflavin, vitamin B_2	0.10 mg	(1%)
Niacin, vitamin B_3	0.20 mg	(1%)
Pantothenic acid, vitamin B_5	0.20 mg	(2%)
Vitamin B_6	0.01 mg	(2%)
Folate, vitamin B_9	8 mcg	(2%)
Vitamin C	29.10 mg	(48%)
Calcium	33 mg	(3%)
Choline	5.10 mg	
Copper	0.10 mg	(3%)
Vitamin E (Alpha Tocopherol)	0.20 mg	(1%)
Electrolytes		
Flavonoids		
Iron	.50 mg	(3%)
Vitamin K	0.60 mcg	(1%)
Magnesium	6 mg	(1%)
Manganese	trace	
Phosphorus	18 mg	(2%)
Potassium	102 mg	(3%)
Selenium	0.40 mcg	(1%)
Zinc	0.10 mg	(1%)
Omega-3 fatty acids	19 mg	
Omega-6 fatty acids	36 mg	
Calories	20	(1%)

Let's look at a bit of what's relevant in these nutrients:

Calorie: The food calorie (as distinguished from the chemistry calorie, which is one-tenth as much) is the energy needed to raise the temperature of one kilogram of water by one degree Celsius.

Carbohydrates: These are the organic compounds, which include sugars, starch, and cellulose. They contain hydrogen and oxygen in the same ratio as water (2:1) and can be broken down to release energy in the body.

Sugars: Sweet crystalline substances from plants such as sugar cane and sugar beet. Sugars are soluble, crystalline, typically sweet-tasting carbohydrates such as glucose and sucrose, found in living tissues. The simple sugar glucose is an important energy source in organisms and is a component of many carbohydrates.

Dietary Fiber: Contains substances such as cellulose, lignin (organic polymer in many plant cell walls), and pectin, which are resistant to the action of digestive enzymes.

Omega-3 & Omega-6 fatty acids: The human body cannot synthesize omega fatty acids, which are necessary for health. They must be acquired through our diet. Omega-3 and omega-6 fatty acids are both short-chain fatty acids that the human body uses to build long-chain fatty acids. Unsaturated fatty acids have been found to prevent heart disease, alleviate depression, reduce inflammation, lower blood pressure, regulate cholesterol levels and reduce risk of blood clot.

Both omega-3 and omega-6 fatty acids are important contributors to normal growth and development and the function of the brain. They stimulate skin and hair growth, regulate metabolism, support healthy bones, and maintain the reproductive system.

Omega-6 fatty acids have proven to reduce symptoms of allergies, high blood pressure, diabetic neuropathy, and rheumatoid arthritis. They are helpful to ease the symptoms of multiple sclerosis, menopause, ADHD, eczema and breast cancer.

Protein: Nitrogen-based, organic compounds of large molecules, composed of one or more long chains of amino acids. These compounds are an essential part of all living organisms, particularly relating to structural components of body tissues such as collagen, hair, muscles, and the like, as well as enzymes and antibodies.

Vitamins and Minerals:

Vitamin A, Retinol: Essential for growth and vision in dim light. A yellow compound found in green and yellow vegetables and in egg yolk.

Thiamine, vitamin B_1: The first water-soluble vitamin "discovered." Originally named aneurin because of the neurological effects that presented if there was no "aneurin" in the diet. However, it was ultimately renamed vitamin B_1. It is used in biosynthesis of gamma-aminobutyric acid (GABA) and the neurotransmitter, acetylcholine.

All living organisms must have thiamine in their diet, but only plants, fungi, and bacteria can synthesize it.

Beriberi, Korsakoff's syndrome, and optic neuropathy result from thiamine deficiency in mammals, with terminal results if not treated. Minor deficiency results in confusion, irritability, weight loss, and/or malaise.

Thiamine derivatives have recently been discovered and are believed to be effective in alleviating impaired glucose metabolism in diabetes.

Riboflavin, vitamin B_2: Riboflavin is required for a variety of cellular processes, including the metabolism of carbohydrates, proteins, fats, and ketone bodies. It's also required by all flavoproteins. Riboflavin is bright yellow and gives B complex pills their coloring.

Niacin, vitamin B$_3$: Also known as nicotinic acid. Niacin contributes to DNA repair and, in the adrenal gland, the production of steroid hormones. A mild niacin deficiency slows metabolism, which results in an intolerance to cold.

A significant niacin deficiency develops into the disease, pellagra, with symptoms of dermatitis, dementia, hyper-pigmentation, tongue and mouth inflammation, lesions on the neck, amnesia, irritability, fatigue, apathy, and depression, and is terminal if not treated.

Pantothenic acid, vitamin B$_5$: A water-soluble vitamin that is an essential nutrient to synthesize and metabolize carbohydrates, fats, and proteins and to synthesize coenzyme-A (CoA). Its name in Greek means "from everywhere," and, indeed, small to large amounts of pantothenic acid is in nearly every food. Pantothenic acid is found in numerous biological actions and is essential to all forms of life. Deficiencies contribute to numerous health concerns and diseases.

Vitamin B$_6$: Butpyridoxal phosphate (PLP), the active form of this water-soluble vitamin, is a cofactor in the reaction of amino acid metabolism. It is also necessary for the enzymatic reaction in the release of glucose from glycogen.

Folate, vitamin B$_9$: Also known as folic acid, vitamin M, vitamin B$_c$ (or folacin), pteroyl-L-glutamic acid, pteroyl-L-glutamate, and pteroylmonoglutamic acid—all forms of the water-soluble vitamin, B_9. After it is converted to dihydrofolic acid in the liver, it becomes important for its derivatives essential to various bodily functions, such as synthesizing DNA, repairing DNA, and to methylate (mix with a methyl group) DNA, which is of particular importance in the rapid cell division of an embryo. Folic acid is required to produce healthy red blood cells and to prevent anemia.

Vitamin C: Citric acid or ascorbic acid is an essential nutrient for humans. It contains a number of vitamers (chemical compounds with similar molecular structures) that produce the activity of vitamin C in animals. These vitamers include ascorbic acid and its salts, as well as oxidized forms of the molecule.

Vitamin C is a primary water-soluble antioxidant in food and the primary water-soluble antioxidant in the body. It is known for supporting cardiovascular health, reducing inflammation, maintaining collagen, aiding in the growth and repair of tissue and the formation of red blood cells.

It contributes to the healing of wounds and ulcers, prevents bleeding from capillaries, and prevents hemorrhaging. Vitamin C helps with calcium metabolism, improves iron absorption, regenerates vitamin

E and converts the inactive form of folic acid into its active, bioavailable, form.

The University of Maryland Medical Center notes that vitamin C deficiency has serious consequences such as stroke, hypertension and gallbladder disease.[9]

Vitamin C is vital to the function of a strong immune system. The high concentration of vitamin C in lemons and limes augments the strength of the immune system, fighting illness and reducing the risk of many diseases, as well as protecting against damage caused by pollution and cigarette smoke.

Vitamin C, also known as L-ascorbic acid, manufactures the body's main protein substance, collagen, and is vital for healthy skin, gums, teeth, blood vessels, tendons, ligaments, cartilage, and bones. Vitamin C heals wounds and reduces scars. It is also an important antioxidant providing protection against free radicals that destroy cells.

Even more amazing than its antioxidant properties is the role of vitamin C in "stereospecific" enzymic reactions. This is when enzymes produce more and specifically needed enzymes.

Vitamin C is a cofactor—which means it must be present for the activity of the enzyme to occur—in at least eight enzymic reactions, including several collagen synthesis reactions. When collagen synthesis reactions are inadequate, the severe symptoms of scurvy soon appear.

Ascorbate is the negatively charged ion, called an "anion," of ascorbic acid. It is necessary for a number of metabolic reactions in all animals and plants. Almost all organisms synthesize vitamin C for themselves. But there are a few exceptions: bats, guinea pigs, capybaras, some species of fish and birds, and one of the two major primate suborders that includes tarsiers, monkeys, apes, and humans.

All species that don't synthesize ascorbate in their bodies must have it in their daily diets. And, once again, in humans, lack of vitamin C quickly erupts with the disease symptoms of scurvy.

When we are under stress, our store of vitamin C rapidly depletes, and the body becomes acidic. Adequate daily intake of vitamin C helps support adrenal gland functions, which in turn assists the body in recovering from stress. It is a circular upward or downward spiral, depending on adequate or inadequate intake of vitamin C.

Free radicals are an endless challenge to a healthy body, and even more so for an unhealthy body. Free radicals ravage healthy cells and damage blood vessels. They change cholesterol so that it deposits plaques of fatty material that builds up on artery walls, eventually becoming atherosclerosis.

Free radicals also cause the painful inflammation and / or swelling of osteoarthritis and rheumatoid arthritis.

Unchecked, free radicals contribute to the development of diabetic heart disease, and many other diseases as well.

Once again, lemons and limes with their high levels of Vitamin C to the rescue! Vitamin C travels through the body, neutralizing free radicals in the aqueous environment, both inside and outside of cells, halting the development of disease in its tracks.

Calcium: Calcium is central to maintaining healthy bones and in regulating the contraction of muscles. (Do you suffer from leg cramps? They will abate if you get enough of the highly bioavailable form of calcium in fresh lemon and lime.) Be sure to supplement with vitamin D, which works to increase the absorption of dietary calcium.

Calcium and magnesium are both plentiful, in good ratio, and are synergistic to each other in lemon or lime juice. Magnesium is important for heart health and calcium prevents rickets.

Choline: Important in the synthesis and transport of lipids. It is a strong, basic compound, found in living tissues.

Copper: A medium-sized lemon has about eight percent of the recommended daily allowance of copper. Copper is found in many of the enzymes that form proteins in the body, including collagen connective protein and the blood's hemoglobin.

Collagen holds tissues and cells together, and hemoglobin protein allows red blood cells to carry oxygen throughout the body.

Vitamin E: This vital vitamin is made up of several fat-soluble alcohol compounds with antioxidant properties that stabilize cell membranes. Vitamin E is also found in leafy vegetables, wheat germ oil, and egg yolks.

Electrolytes: Ionized or ionizable components of blood, a living cell, or other organic matter.

Flavonoids: These are plant pigment crystalline compounds. They have numerous positive aspects including antioxidant and anticancer properties. Lemon and lime flavonoids are called *flavonol glycosides*, and include a number of *kaempferol*-related molecules.

These flavonoids have been shown to stop cell division in many cancer cell lines, and are also very interesting for their antibiotic effects. Flavonoids enhance the numerous functions of vitamin C.

The flavonoid limonene has anticancer effects. It increases the level of enzymes that detoxify carcinogens. Lemons and limes are full of bioflavonoid antioxidant phytonutrients (also known as vitamin P).

Kaempferol and some glycosides of kaempferol have a wide range of pharmacological processes including: cardio-protective, neuro-protective, anti-osteoporotic, anti-diabetic, anxiolytic (substances that reduce anxiety), and are both estrogenic and anti-estrogenic (yes! In other words, these substances promote the appropriate amount of estrogen in women and interfere with estrogen-production in men).

Again, the flavonoids have antioxidant, anti-inflammatory, antimicrobial, anticancer, antibacterial, antibiotic (distinct from antibacterial due to the newly developed and being developed antimicrobial compounds and anti-fungal compounds) analgesic, and antiallergic activities.

Epidemiological studies have found a positive link between eating foods containing kaempferol and a reduced risk of developing cardiovascular diseases or cancer.

Iron: An essential mineral that transports oxygen throughout the body. A slight deficiency of iron causes anemia, with its attendant fatigue and weakness. A chronic iron deficiency can lead to organ failure.

Lemons and limes are a good source of iron, plus their vitamin C increases the absorption of iron.

Vitamin K: A group of vitamins found mainly in green leaves, such as cabbage and spinach. Vitamin K_1 and vitamin K_2 are essential for the blood-clotting process.

Magnesium: Important for heart health. As noted above, synergistic with calcium. In terms of its mass, magnesium is the eleventh most abundant element in the human body. Magnesium ions manipulate the polyphosphate compounds of DNA, RNA, and ATP (adenosine triphosphate). Therefore, enzymes are dependent upon magnesium ions to function properly.

Manganese: This element is a required trace mineral for living organisms. The enzymes of manganese are essential to detox superoxide free radicals.

Phosphorus: Essential for life, it is a component of DNA, RNA, and ATP. Cell membranes are formed of phospholipids.

Potassium: Lemons and limes rate high for their amount of potassium. This electrolytic mineral is crucial in regulating the activity of the cells in your body. Potassium helps to maintain the proper balance of fluid in tissues and cells. Lemons and limes are rich in potassium citrate, which becomes two important alkalizing substances, potassium and bicarbonate, when metabolized in your body.

Sodium and potassium work together to produce the electrical transmissions in your nervous system, brain and heart to keep a steady flow of electrical impulses.

Forgetfulness, anxiety, fogginess, and depression are frequently traced to inadequate potassium blood levels.

Proteins: Nitrogenous organic compounds consisting of large molecules, composed of one or more long chains of amino acids. They are an essential part of all living organisms.

Selenium: A trace mineral essential to good health. It is incorporated into proteins to make the antioxidant enzymes, selenoproteins. Some selenoproteins help prevent cellular damage from free radicals, and others build up the immune system or help regulate the thyroid.

Zinc: An essential mineral. Deficiency of zinc is a huge concern in the developing world, affecting two billion people. Eight-hundred-thousand children die every year from zinc deficiency, which retards growth and causes susceptibility to infections, diseases, and chronic diarrhea.

It's believed by people who have taken zinc supplements that it restores gray hair to its natural color (although excess zinc can have serious negative repercussions such as lethargy, ataxia and copper deficiency).

Energy from Food—Atoms & Molecules

The energy from food comes from its atoms and molecules. An ion is part of a molecule that carries either a negative or positive electrical charge. In their atomic structure, lemons and limes have more negatively charged ions, called "anions," than positively charged ions, called "cations."

Much of our diet is cationic—it has a positive charge and is acidic. Food is turned into fuel or energy when it encounters saliva (which can range from acidic to alkaline), hydrochloric acid (a strong acid) and bile (alkaline) and the stomach's other digestive juices, and the digestive processes occur.

Lemon and lime juice assists in the digestive process. Because lemons and limes are very low sugar fruits, their acids are readily metabolized to sodium bicarbonate, a base, (negative charge) alkaline substance. The few cations (positively charged acids) in lemons and limes are entirely offset by the sodium bicarbonate, netting an anionic, negative charge, alkaline result, contributing to the much-needed alkalizing balance.

IMPORTANT NOTE: Any form of packaged lemon or lime juice (frozen, fresh frozen, bottled) is cationic (acidic) by virtue of the processing, and is not effective as a health remedy in the sense that anionic (alkaline), fresh squeezed lemon or lime juice is.

More Information about Antioxidants

An antioxidant is a molecule that keeps other molecules from becoming oxidized. This is good because when the molecules we need become oxidized, they produce free radicals, and the free radicals, like a gang of outlaws, start chain reactions that damage or kill healthy cells.

Enter the white hat guys, the antioxidants, *which are themselves* oxidized and act as reducing agents on the free radicals so that they can no longer commit mayhem and murder. Ascorbic acid and polyphenols are antioxidants.

More Information about Enzymes

Cells make enzymes. Enzymes are protein catalysts that provide a surface, that is to say, a stage upon which the reactants, which are any of the substances that undergo a change during a reaction, can come together in their proper orientation. Enzymes are very specific and only particular reactants will fit on the active site of their surface. A set of reactants for an enzyme is called its substrate.

Catalysts—including enzymes—are not changed by the reaction they cause. So, after all the reactants have been converted to their useful and necessary components, the enzyme molecule remains. However, the environment of the enzyme is critical for the enzyme to be able to do its job. This is yet another reason why balanced pH is so vitally important, as enzymes cannot thrive in an acidic environment.

NOTE: A food's acid content doesn't determine its pH nature in your body. It's the metabolic process that affects whether a food primarily contributes acidic or alkaline substances to your body. As mentioned elsewhere, lemons and limes burn as alkaline ash in the body, rendering their process as alkaline.

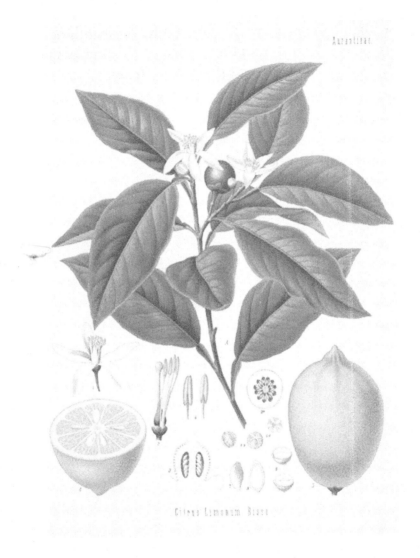

Chapter 8:
Concerns & Cautions

"If you do just one thing that can change the world, buy organic food ... No other single choice you can make to improve the health of your family and the planet will have greater positive repercussions for our future."

Maria Rodale,
Organic Manifesto

Here are a few concerns, followed by the cautions that are found throughout the book, placed together for easy reference.

Lemons and Limes and Wax Coatings

Lemons and limes are sometimes coated to protect them during shipping. The coatings may be animal, insect, plant or petroleum-based, with carnauba palm being the most common. Ethyl alcohol, ethanol, milk casein or soaps may be added to the wax. So, once again, it's suggested that you soak your produce in room temperature water with a tablespoon of sea salt for ten minutes when you get home. Also, scrub the fruit before cutting it to be sure wax residue has been removed. Buy organic when you can.

Not Recommended

As mentioned, frozen or bottled, reconstituted lemon and lime juice is *NOT* the same as fresh-squeezed juice. It has been processed and contains preservatives, (for example, Sodium Bisulfite and Sodium Benzoate).

The particular powerhouse of lemon and lime juice is the delicate enzymes, antioxidants, biophotons, and phytonutrients, which are almost certainly no longer active in reconstituted, bottled or frozen juice.

Preservatives are acidic and do not burn to alkaline ash. The reconstituted lemon or lime juice still has vitamins and minerals, but otherwise, it does not compare with fresh-squeezed juice.

Given that the vitamins and minerals remain, it is definitely better than nothing. If you're traveling or otherwise removed from fresh lemons and limes, do continue to have your daily lemon or lime tonic with bottled juice, but get the fresh fruit when and wherever you can. If you go to a restaurant, ask for a small dish of lemon slices. I've never been refused this request. Granted, they've already been sliced and exposed to air (unless you can convince your kind wait person to bring you a half-a-lemon!).

Even though there is a small amount of preservatives in the reconstituted juice, you need to be aware that the preservatives are there. Some people have a reaction to very small amounts. In any case, if something is an allergen to an individual, how little is "just a little?"

Cautions

People on blood thinners, please discuss your intention to begin a regime of daily consumption of lemon and/or lime juice with your health care professional.

Some people are allergic to citrus peels, so when you consume lime or lemon juice extracted together with the peel, check yourself to see if there is any allergic reaction.

Straight lemon or lime juice can be harmful to the enamel of your teeth. Mix the juice with water or follow with a glass of water.

DO NOT IGNORE gallbladder discomfort. You *MUST* get medical attention for your gallbladder issues. A ruptured gallbladder is life-threatening. If a gallbladder ruptures, it must be removed. The remedies suggested in this book are for prevention.

Although there are many benefits to eating the peel of lemons and limes, they do contain oxalates, and oxalates can crystallize. People who tend to have kidney stones, pancreatic stones, or gallstones should avoid eating lemon or lime peel and be aware of foods with lemon or lime zest.

All things in moderation. It is possible, but extremely unlikely in our overly acidic environment, diet and lifestyle, to become over-alkaline.

Make sure to rinse lemon juice off of your skin before you go out into the sun. The juice will increase your skin's sensitivity to UV rays (unless you are under specific treatment for your skin).

DO NOT neglect or put off going to the dentist if you have a toothache or other dental problem.

There are certain cautions regarding taking medications with grapefruit juice, and as lemons and limes are similar to grapefruit and have similar behaviors in the body, it's advised to drink your lemon or lime juice an hour away from taking medications. Always check this information out with your health care practitioner.

GLOSSARY:

Acetylcholine - A neuro-transmitting compound found throughout the nervous system.

Acidic - pH below 7.

Albedo - The white pith of citrus fruit.

Alkaline - pH greater than 7.

Allergens - Substances causing allergic reactions.

Antibiotic - A substance that inhibits the growth of or destroys microorganisms.

Antibodies - Blood proteins that are produced in response to, and counteracting, an antigen. Antibodies combine chemically with substances the body recognizes as alien such as bacteria, viruses, and foreign substances in the blood to destroy them and keep the body healthy.

Antibacterial - A substance or process that is active against bacteria.

Anti-fungal - A substance or process that is active against fungus.

Antihistamine - A compound for treating allergies that inhibits the effects of histamine.

Anti-inflammatory - Used to reduce inflammation.

Antioxidants - A substance such as vitamin C or E that removes potentially damaging oxidizing agents in a living organism.

Antiseptic - Substances that prevent the growth of disease-causing microorganisms.

Antiviral - A substance or process that is effective against viruses.

Apo B - The structural protein of the LDL cholesterol molecule.

Ayurvedic/Ayurveda - East Indian ancient and present-day medicine.

Bile - A bitter greenish-brown alkaline fluid that aids digestion. It is secreted by the liver and stored in the gallbladder.

Bioavailable - A substance that enters circulation when introduced into the body and is able to have an active effect.

Biophotons - The name comes from the Greek words for "light" and "life." A biophoton is a photon of light in the ultraviolet and visible spectrum that is emitted from a biological form. This includes lemons, limes, and *you!*

Biosynthesis - The production of complex molecules in living organisms or cells.

Carcinogenic - Having the potential to cause cancer.

Catalyst - A substance that increases the rate of a chemical reaction without itself changing.

Chelator - A molecule that binds to another, usually larger, molecule.

Cholesterol - A sterol compound found in most body tissues including blood and nerves.

Cholesterol and its derivatives are important components of cell membranes. They are precursors of other steroid compounds. However, high concentrations in the blood, derived from animal fats in the diet, are believed to promote atherosclerosis.

LDL - bad - the form of lipoprotein in which cholesterol is transported in the blood.

HDL - good - high-density lipoprotein that removes cholesterol from the blood. It is associated with a reduced risk of atherosclerosis and heart disease.

Citric acid - The primary carrier of biochemicals in the body.

Citron - The fruit of a small, thorny evergreen tree that grows 8 to 15 feet tall, native to India and Southeast Asia. Its molecular structure provides evidence that our cultivated citrus came from developing hybrids of the citron.

Electrolytes - The ionized or ionizable components of blood, a living cell, or other organic matter.

Enzymes - Substances produced by a living organism that act as catalysts to bring about specific biochemical reactions. Most enzymes are proteins of large, complex molecules. Their action depends on their particular molecular shape. Some enzymes, such as the enzymes involved in digestion, control reactions outside of cells, and some enzymes control reactions within cells.

Flavanone - From flavone, crystalline and colorless.

Flavone - A tricyclic, aromatic compound that is colorless and crystalline and is the basis of a number of white or yellow plant pigments.

Flavonoids - Plant pigments that have a structure based on a flavone.

Free radicals - A very unstable molecule, which is missing an electron. A free radical will react quickly with other compounds to capture an electron, attacking the nearest stable molecule. Then that molecule becomes a free radical, thus triggering a chain reaction that can destroy a living cell.

Gamma-aminobutyric acid (GABA) - Biochemical process. An amino acid that inhibits the transmission of nerve impulses in the central nervous system.

Glycemic index - Foods are ranked on a scale from 1 to 100 based on their effect on blood sugar levels.

Hypertension - High blood pressure.

Kaempferol - A flavonoid in the oil of lemons and limes.

Lactic acid - A colorless organic acid formed in sour milk and produced in muscle tissues during strenuous exercise. Trace amounts are found in lemons and limes.

Limonene - Extremely bioavailable, disease-fighting, compounds.

Limonins - An extremely bioavailable limonoid. It is white, crystalline, and bitter-tasting, found in citrus and other plants.

Limonoids - Extremely bioavailable, disease-fighting, compounds and potent anti-carcinogens.

Lipids - Fats - A class of organic compounds that are fatty acids, or their derivatives. They are not soluble in water but are soluble in organic solvents.

Macromolecules - Food broken down into usable components. A molecule containing a very large number of atoms, such as a protein or nucleic acid.

Microorganisms - A microscopic organism, such as a bacterium, virus, or fungus.

Naringenin - An antioxidant, a free radical scavenger, and an anti-inflammatory flavanone.

Neurotransmitter - A chemical substance that is released at the end of a nerve fiber during a nerve impulse, diffusing across the synapse and causing the transfer of the impulse to another nerve fiber, a muscle fiber, or other structure.

Nitrosamines - Carcinogenic chemical compounds.

Nutrients - Any substance, such as protein, vitamins, or minerals that provide nourishment for the growth and maintenance of life.

Oxalates - Crystalline acid with a sour taste, present in rhubarb leaves, wood sorrel, and other plants, including the peel of lemons and limes.

Oxidize - The action of substances becoming combined chemically with oxygen. A chemical reaction in which electrons are lost.

Pathogenic - A bacterium, virus, or other microorganism that can cause disease.

Pectin - A soluble gelatinous polysaccharide, a carbohydrate (e.g., starch, cellulose, or glycogen) whose molecules consist of a number of sugar molecules bonded together, present in ripe fruits. Extracted for use as a setting agent in jams and jellies.

pH scale - A scale measuring from one, which is extremely acidic, to fourteen, which is extremely alkaline.

pH balance - The need for every living thing to maintain a balanced pH near 7.365 on the pH scale.

Phytochemicals - The chemistry of plants and plant products.

Phytonutrients - A plant substance that has nutritional value, or a nutritional supplement, known as a nutraceutical.

Psoralens - A group of chemical compounds found in particular plants that are used in the treatment of psoriasis and vitiligo.

Purines - Metabolized chemicals that form uric acid on oxidation.

Reactants - the substances that take part in, and that undergo, change during a reaction.

Siddha - East Indian ancient and present-day medicine.

Soluble - Able to be dissolved, particularly in water.

Toxins - Harmful chemicals.

Uric acid - Derived from purines. When uric acid crystallizes it becomes gout.

Uricase - A digestive enzyme that breaks down purines.

Urinary citrate - Can prevent and even cure the mineral crystallization that makes kidney stones, pancreatic stones, and gallstones.

Zest - The peel of lemons and limes ground up for cooking and as a garnish.

Footnotes:

1. Dr. Alexander F. Beddoe, *Biological Ionization as Applied to Human Nutrition* (Wendell Whitman Co. June 2002)

2. *The Journal of Urology*; American Urological Association, Linthicum, MD
http://www.auanet.org/content/homepage/homepage.cfm

3. *Nutrition and Cancer* (Taylor & Francis/Routledge, Philadelphia, PA. 2001/2009/2012)
http://www.tandfonline.com/

4. *Annals of the Rheumatic Diseases* (BMA House, London, UK)
http://ard.bmj.com/

5. *Effects of Limonene and Essential Oil from Citrus Aurantium on Gastric Mucosa: Role of Prostaglandins and Gastric Mucus Secretion; Chemico-biological Interactions*, São Paulo State University, Department of Physiology, São Paulo, Brazil Aug 14, 2009; 180(3): 499-505/Epub 2009 May 3
http://www.ncbi.nlm.nih.gov/pubmed/19410566#

6. The Linus Pauling Institute, Oregon State University, 307 Linus Pauling Science Center, Corvallis, Oregon
http://lpi.oregonstate.edu/

7. *Colorless Tetrapyrrolic Chlorophyll Catabolites Found in Ripening Fruit are Effective Antioxidants*; Institute of Organic Chemistry & Centre for Molecular Biosciences Innsbruck, University of Innsbruck, Innsbruck, Austria, Agnew Chem Int. Ed., 2007; Nov. 46(45) :8699-702
http://www.ncbi.nlm.nih.gov/pubmed?Db=pubmed&Cmd=ShowDetailView&TermToSearch=17943948&ordinalpos=1&itool=EntrezSystem2.PEntrez.Pubmed.Pubmed_ResultsPanel.Pubmed_RVDocSum

8. ibid.

9. The University of Maryland Medical Center, 22 S Greene St, Baltimore, MD.
http://www.umm.edu/

References & Resources:

Internet:

Does Vitamin C Make the Body More Acidic?
http://www.livestrong.com/article/549473-vitamin-c-make-body-acidic/

Fibrotalk–Support and Information
http://www.fibrotalk.com/forum/viewtopic.php?f=90&t=28778

Health Benefits of Lemon Water
http://www.marcussamuelsson.com/recipe/recipe-health-benefits-of-lemon-water

Health Benefits of Lime
http://www.organicfacts.net/health-benefits/fruit/health-benefits-of-lime.html

National Center for Biotechnology Information
http://www.ncbi.nlm.nih.gov/

Raw Limes–Nutrition Chart–Self.com
http://nutritiondata.self.com/facts/fruits-and-fruit-juices/1942/2#ixzz2N6wVqNXC

Raw Lemons–Nutrition Chart–Self.com
http://nutritiondata.self.com/facts/fruits-and-fruit-juices/1936/2

The Difference Between Citric Acid, Ascorbic Acid & Sorbic Acid
http://www.livestrong.com/article/170330-the-difference-between-citric-acid-ascorbic-acid-sorbic-acid/#ixzz2L6vkJwWq

University of Maryland Medical Center–Omega 6 Fatty Acids
http://www.umm.edu/altmed/articles/omega-6-000317.htm#ixzz2Nd1sG32d

University of Maryland Medical Center–Omega 3 Fatty Acids
http://www.umm.edu/altmed/articles/omega-3-000316.htm

U.S. Food and Drug Administration's Reference Values for Nutrition Labeling
http://www.nutrition.gov/shopping-cooking-meal-planning/food-labels

Wikipedia: numerous and sundry references. *Thank you, Wiki.*

Books & Journals:

Berhow MA, Bennett RD, Poling SM, et al. *Acylated Flavonoids in Callus Cultures of Citrus aurantifolia.* Phytochemistry 1994 July 36 (5):1225-7. 1994.

Cheung, Theresa; *The Lemon Juice Diet*, St. Martin's Paperbacks; First Edition, April 27, 2010.

Gharagozloo M, Ghaderi A. *Immunomodulatory Effect of Concentrated Lime Juice Extract on Activated Human Mononuclear Cells.* Journal of Ethnopharmacolgy 2001 Sept 77 (1):85-90. 2001.

Kawaii S, Tomono Y, Katase E, et al. *Antiproliferative Effects of the Readily Extractable Fractions Prepared from Various Citrus Juices on Several Cancer Cell Lines.* Journal of Agricultural Food Chemistry 1999 July 47(7):2509-12. 1999.

Kloss, Jethro; *Back to Eden*, Back to Eden Publishing, by Lotus Press, Twin Lakes, WI, Revised Edition (January 22, 2004) 936 pages.

Kurl S, Tuomainen TP, Laukkanen JA et al. *Plasma Vitamin C Modifies the Association Between Hypertension and Risk of Stroke.* Stroke 2002 June 33(6):1568-73. 2002.

Pattison DJ, Silman AJ, Goodson NJ, Lunt M, Bunn D, Luben R, Welch A, Bingham S, Khaw KT, Day N,

Symmons DP. *Vitamin C and the Risk of Developing Inflammatory Polyarthritis: Prospective Nested Case-Control Study*. Ann Rheum Dis. 2004 July 63 (7):843-7. 2004.

Popp, F.A., Gu, Q. and Li, K.H.: *Biophoton Emission: Experimental Background and Theoretical Approaches.* Modern Physics Letters B, Vol.8, Nos. 21 & 22 (1994), pp.1269-1296.

Rodrigues A, Sandstrom A, Ca T, *et al. Protection from Cholera by Adding Lime Juice to Food - Community and Laboratory Studies in Guinea-Bissau, West Africa.* Tropical Med Int Health 2000 June 5 (6):418-22. 2000.

DISCLAIMER:

Any medically related content is not intended to be medical advice or instructions for medical diagnosis or treatment. If you think you may have a medical emergency, call your doctor or your local emergency number immediately. This information is not a substitute for professional medical advice, examination, diagnosis, or treatment. Do not delay or forego seeking treatment for a medical condition or disregard professional medical advice based on any content herein. Always seek the advice of your physician or other qualified healthcare professional before starting or changing any treatment.

My Gift for You ....

As a thank you for reading *Save Your Live with the Phenomenal Lemon & Lime*, I have a gift for you, *Save Your Life with Stupendous Spices*. To receive your ebook, type in the following link:

https://BookHip.com/DKHVDA

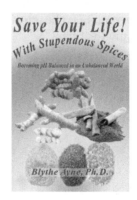

About the Author

I live in a forest with a few domestic and numerous wild creatures, where I create an ever-growing inventory of books, both nonfiction and fiction, short stories, illustrated kid's books, and articles, with a bit of wood carving when I need a change of pace.

I received my Doctorate from the University of California at Irvine in the School of Social Sciences, majoring in psychology and ethnography, after which I moved to the Pacific Northwest to write and to have a modest private psychotherapy practice in a small town not much bigger than a village. Finally I decided it was time to put my full focus on my writing, where, through the world-shrinking internet, I could "meet" greater numbers of people. Where I could meet you!

All the creatures in my forest and I thank you for "stopping by. If *Save Your Life with the Phenomenal Lemon & Lime* has touched you in a positive way I hope you'll consider writing a review, as reviews are an author's life's blood, as well as an excellent means for people to discover books that might inspire them on their way.

I Wish You Happiness, Health, Peace, and Joy,
Blythe

Questions or observations? I'd love to hear from you!

Blythe@BlytheAyne.com

www.BlytheAyne.com

15.
17.

Made in the USA
Las Vegas, NV
06 November 2022

58843619R00085